D1135220

Ambulance:

Fire:

Police:

Taxi services: telephone

Dentist

Address

Telephone

Other specialists and consultants

Person to contact in emergency

Address

Telephone

The Pocket Medical and First Aid Guide

Emergencies Symptoms Treatments

Dr James Bevan
MA, MB, BChir, MRCGP, DObst. RCOG

Mitchell Beazley

Advisory Panel

R. W. Beard, MD, FRCOG,
Professor of Obstetrics and Gynaecology,
St Mary's Hospital, London

A. W. Boylston, MD, MRCPath,
Wellcome Senior Fellow in Clinical Science,
St Mary's Hospital Medical School, London

Anthony Catterall, MChir, FRCS,
Consultant Orthopaedic Surgeon,
Royal National Orthopaedic Hospital
and New Charing Cross Hospital, London

Dr R.M. Moffitt, MA, MB, MRCP, MRCGP, DO,
General Practitioner and Senior
Medical Officer, University of Lancaster

Dr J.F. Robinson, MB, ChB, MRCGP,
General Practitioner

The Pocket Medical and First Aid Guide
was edited and designed by Mitchell Beazley Publishers Limited,
87-89 Shaftesbury Avenue, London W1V 7AD

© Mitchell Beazley Publishers Limited 1979
Text © Fennlevel Limited 1979
All rights reserved

Reprinted 1979, 1980, 1981, 1982, 1983
ISBN 0 85533 151 8

Printed & bound in Great Britain

Contents

Editor
Hal Robinson
Editorial Assistants
Rosemary Bevan
Melita Brownrigg
Margaret Butcher
Joyce Evison
Sarah Gratton
Cynthia Hole
Valerie Nicholson
Janet Proffitt

Art Editor
John Ridgeway
Designer
Piers Evelegh
Artists
David Ashby
Priscilla Barrett
Terry Lawler
Coral Mula
Production
Graham Darlow

Emergency First Aid

Introduction

When an emergency occurs and there is no doctor present it is important to do the right thing as quickly and as calmly as possible. The chart on the opposite page shows the steps you must take. These may save the patient's life if it is in danger. Ways to treat the most serious emergencies are described on pp.5-17. Advice about treating children in emergencies is given on pp.18-19.

Index to Emergency First Aid

Index to First Aid Techniques

Other emergency situations, and the ways to deal with them, are described on pp.20-35. See the index below:

Survival Techniques. See pp.36-40

First Aid at an Accident

CALL FOR HELP. IF THE CASUALTY'S NECK IS BROKEN, DO NOT DISTURB

⬇

CHECK FOR BREATHING (p.6)

⬇ ⬇

BREATHING | **NOT BREATHING**

⬇ ⬇

OBSERVE. IF NO FRACTURES (p.11) PLACE IN RECOVERY POSITION (p.12). CHECK FOR BLEEDING (p.10) | **CLEAR AIRWAY (p.7)**

CHECK FOR A PULSE (p.6)

⬇ ⬇

PULSE | **NO PULSE**

⬇ ⬇

GIVE ARTIFICIAL RESPIRATION (p.9) | **GIVE HEART MASSAGE AND ARTIFICIAL RESPIRATION (p.9)**

⬇

CONTINUE UNTIL HEARTBEAT AND RESPIRATION START AGAIN

In all cases the casualty must lie on the floor

If **bleeding**	— press on source of bleeding	p.10
If **bones fractured**	— do not move the casualty	p.11
If **burned**, by fire	— soak with cold water	p.10
If **burned**, by liquids	— remove soaked clothes	p.10
If **choking**	— force air out of the lungs	p.13
If **conscious**	— keep the casualty talking	p.12
If having **convulsions**	— do not restrict movement	p.14
If **poisoned** or **stung**	— keep the casualty calm	p.15
If **unconscious**	— check pulse and breathing	p.12

Checking for Breathing and Pulse

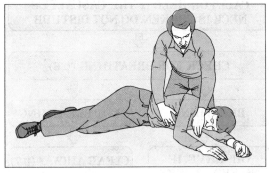

1. Check for breathing. *Feel for breathing by placing your hand on the casualty's* chest and in front of the mouth and nose. Always call for medical assistance.

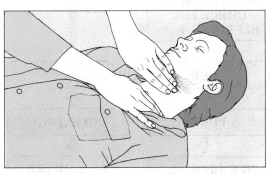

2. Check for a pulse. *The strongest pulse is in the neck. It can be felt between the* windpipe and the angle of the jaw. The pulse in the wrist is hard to detect.

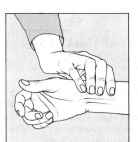

3. Radial pulse. *Hold your fingers on the inside of the wrist in line with the thumb.*

The carotid pulse in the neck gives the clearest indication that the heart is beating. It is often impossible to feel any pulse at all in the wrist of an injured person. The colour and feel of the casualty's skin are other signs of cardiac arrest. The skin is likely to be grey and cold and the lips pale. If the heart is not beating, the casualty needs heart massage at once.

6

Clearing the Airway

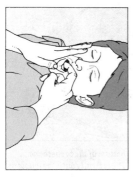

4. Clear the airway and remove anything blocking the free flow of air.

The casualty must be turned face up. Remove obstructions from the mouth by tilting the head to one side and holding the mouth open with your thumb. Use your other hand to remove anything, such as false teeth or a toy, that blocks the casualty's throat. If the mouth is damaged, make sure that the nose is clear so that mouth-to-nose artificial respiration can be used. If this is not possible, see the Silvester or Holger Nielsen methods, pp. 14-15.

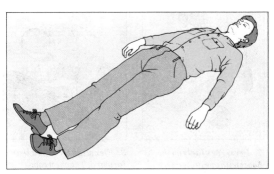

5. Lay casualty face up on a hard surface such as the floor for both heart massage and mouth-to-mouth artificial respiration. Loosen clothing around the neck.

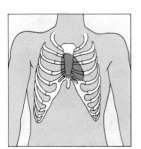

6. The heart lies beneath the breastbone and toward the left of the casualty's chest.

If the casualty's heart has stopped, three quick, firm presses on the chest over the breastbone may start it beating again. If not, a steady, regular rhythm of one press a second is required. This must be continued until the heart starts again or until medical help arrives. Kneel at the casualty's left shoulder and press the chest over the whole area of the heart.

Heart Massage

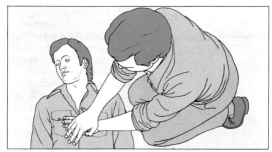

1. Heart massage. Kneel at the casualty's left shoulder. Place one hand on the other so that your fingers touch the bottom of the breastbone. Press firmly with the whole of your hand evenly over the area of the heart.

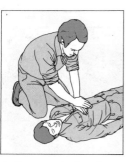

2. Press regularly on the heart with one press a second until the heart starts to beat rhythmically again.

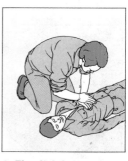

3. Flex slightly as you lean forward. The chest compresses about two inches. For children do not press too hard.

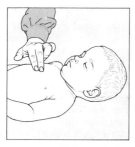

4. For a baby's heart, it is sufficient to press with two fingers only, at about one hundred beats a minute.

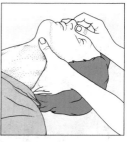

5. Prepare for mouth-to-mouth resuscitation by lifting the casualty's neck, tilting the head and pinching the nose.

Mouth-to-mouth Resuscitation

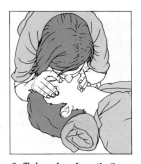

6. Take a deep breath. *Cover the casualty's mouth or nose with your mouth. Blow steadily into the lungs.*

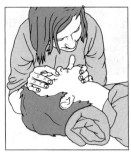

7. Watch the chest fall *as you take another deep breath. If this fails to happen, check that the airway is clear.*

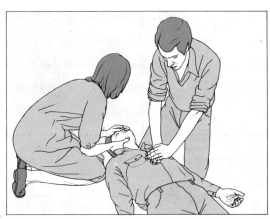

8. Cardio-pulmonary resuscitation. *If the heart has stopped, then breathing will also cease. In this case it is necessary to combine heart massage with mouth-to-mouth artificial respiration. To do this, one person kneels at the casualty's left shoulder to give heart massage at a rate of one press a second. The other kneels at the casualty's right side to give mouth-to-mouth resuscitation as described. You should inflate the chest once every five seconds.*

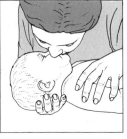

9. For a child or a baby, *cover both mouth and nose with your mouth. Be very careful not to blow too hard.*

Burns and Bleeding

Burns

Burns may be caused by fire, hot water or chemicals. If the casualty's clothes are burning, put out the fire with cold water or by rolling the casualty in a rug, blanket or coat. Leave the burned clothes in place as these will be sterile. Cold water also stops burning by hot water and dilutes corrosive chemicals. Clothing soaked by chemicals must be removed. A burned area of the body should be covered with a dry sterile dressing. The casualty will be suffering from shock, and should lie in the recovery position until medical help arrives (see p.12).

Bleeding

Bleeding must be stopped as quickly as possible. Press hard with your fingers or hand for 20 minutes. If it has not stopped, keep pressing for another 20 minutes.

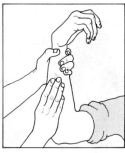

1. For a small wound, press hard with your fingers to stop the blood flow.

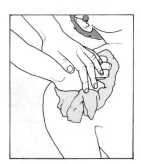

2. For a large wound, use a piece of clean cloth and press hard so that bleeding stops.

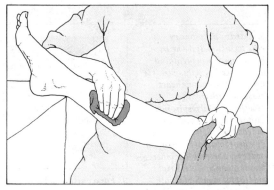

3. For varicose veins, which may bleed profusely if cut, raise the casualty's leg and
press on the site of the bleeding until professional medical assistance arrives.

Fractures

Shock after bleeding and burns

Any seriously injured person suffers from shock. Shock is particularly dangerous if the casualty has suffered burns or blood-loss. In all cases, keep the casualty still, lying in the recovery position if unconscious (see p.12) or lying on the back with the feet raised if conscious. Cover with a blanket and encourage the casualty to talk. If the casualty is unconscious, observe pulse and breathing.

Fractures

As a general rule, do not move the casualty if there is any possibility that bones have been fractured. Moving a fractured limb may cause internal damage, and disturbing a fractured neck may kill the casualty. If someone with a fractured limb must be moved, the limb must be completely immobilized.

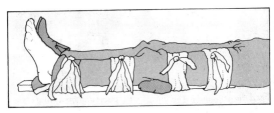

Immobilizing a limb. *A splint is required to prevent the limb moving. With the limb straight, tie a rigid support to the limb. Do not tie at the site of the injury.*

Moving a casualty

Two people can move a casualty safely only with a stretcher. Otherwise a minimum of three people are required.

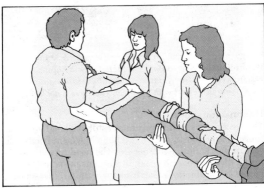

Three-person lift. *For moving an immobilized casualty, one person supports the shoulders and head; a second supports the hips; and a third supports the legs.*

Recovery Position

Recovery position
This is the position in which an unconscious person can breathe most easily.

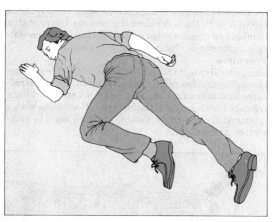

Turn the face *to one side and bend the arm and leg on that same side. The other arm and* *leg should be straight. Check the pulse and breathing every minute.*

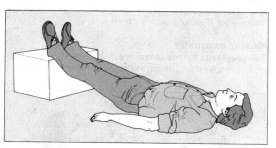

*A **conscious person** recovers best from shock or from fainting by lying on the back with* *the feet raised. Encourage the casualty to talk so that consciousness is not lost.*

Unconsciousness
This occurs most commonly as a result of a head injury. If there is any possibility that a bone has been fractured, and in particular if the neck or the head have been injured, do not move the casualty because this may cause more serious damage. Call a doctor or ambulance as soon as possible. If an unconscious person has difficulty breathing, move this person to the recovery position and check pulse and breathing every minute. The recovery position is also best for someone whose breathing is normal.

Shock and Choking

Shock

The symptoms of shock are a pale skin, restlessness, confusion, anxiety, rapid pulse and shallow rapid breathing. These symptoms are caused by the physical reaction of the body to a traumatic event such as an injury, heart attack, bleeding, burns, extreme or prolonged cold (exposure) or fear. The body reacts by reducing the blood supply to the skin, arms and legs so that an adequate supply to the vital organs (brain, heart, and lungs) can be maintained. A person in shock should lie down, because this helps blood flow to the brain, and should be covered with blankets to reduce heat loss. Do not give extra warmth, alcohol, or hot drinks, as this dilates peripheral blood vessels and takes blood from the vital organs. Consciousness may fluctuate so try to keep the casualty conscious by talking, and observe the pulse and breathing at all times. Keep the person lying as still as possible and call a doctor or an ambulance. Stay with the casualty until recovery from shock is complete. Anyone who is suffering from shock should be kept under medical observation for at least one hour.

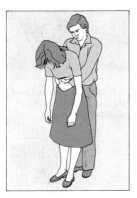

Heimlich manoeuvre.
Hold one hand in the other
and pull sharply upwards.

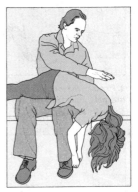

For a child, hold the head
lower than the chest and hit
between the shoulder blades.

Choking

When a person chokes, the blocked air passage must be cleared immediately. When an adult starts to choke, grasp the victim from behind. Clench one hand below the bottom of the rib cage (over the midriff) and hold this clenched hand with the other hand. Pull the hands sharply upwards so that victim's lungs are compressed and the air expelled forcibly from them. This process, the Heimlich manoeuvre, is intended to dislodge the blockage. Artifical respiration may also be required.

13

Artificial Respiration

Convulsions and fits

Do not try to restrict the movements of a person who is having convulsions. Move furniture and other hard objects away from the victim to avoid the danger of these injuring the victim. When the fit has passed leave the victim in the recovery position to rest or sleep.

Artificial respiration

Mouth-to-mouth artificial respiration is the most effective method for restarting breathing. If the mouth and nose are damaged it is not practicable, however, and in such cases the Holger Nielsen or Silvester methods should be used.

Holger Nielsen method

The casualty must be lying face-down. Kneel at the head and lean over so that your hands rest on the casualty's shoulder blades.

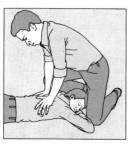

1. Press on the shoulder blades to expel the air from the casualty's lungs.

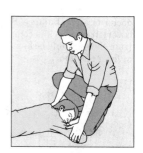

2. Rock backwards and hold the casualty's elbows. Raise these from the ground.

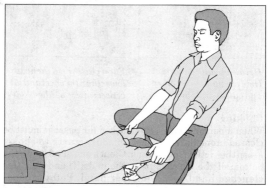

3. Lift the casualty's elbows so that the chest expands and sucks in air.

4. Lower the elbows, and repeat the cycle once every five seconds.

Poisoning and Snakebite

The Silvester method

This is used when the casualty is lying face-up. Heart massage can be given at the same time. To do this, press firmly on the heart once a second when the casualty's arms are raised. One person can combine heart massage with artificial respiration if ten presses on the heart are given between each cycle of the Silvester method, but the combination is easier with two people.

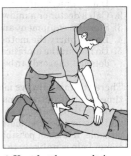

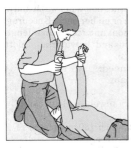

1. Kneel at the casualty's head, hold the wrists and press on the rib cage.

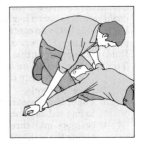

2. Raise the arms upwards and bring them outwards and down by your side.

3. This expands the lungs and sucks air in. Repeat the cycle every five seconds.

Poisoning

In all cases identify the poison and call for medical help immediately. If the poison has been swallowed it can be diluted by giving the victim large quantities of water or milk to drink. Encourage vomiting in all cases unless you are sure the poison is corrosive (acid, alkali, petrol or fuel oil). A solution of salt and sodium bicarbonate in water will cause the victim to vomit. Take a sample of the poison to hospital. Observe the victim's pulse and breathing carefully.

Snakebite

Identify the snake. Kill it if possible and take it with the victim to hospital. Calm the patient because the victim of a snakebite often suffers more seriously from shock than from the poison. Wash the bite thoroughly and immobilize the bitten part. Treat spider bites as snakebites.

Bites

Treat animal bites as open wounds (see p.10), and seek medical advice as soon as possible.

Emergency Childbirth

1. Don't panic. Childbirth is a natural process.
2. Call a doctor or a midwife.
3. Sterilize equipment and wash hands thoroughly.
4. Do not hurry the mother. Let her set the pace.
5. Do not cut the umbilical cord. If medical help is delayed, the cord can be tied.

There is almost always more than half an hour from the time that the contractions of the first stage of labour start to the birth of the baby, so if labour begins, call a doctor or midwife or take the mother to a hospital as quickly as possible. If it is not possible to get to a hospital and professional help is unlikely to arrive in time, find somewhere warm, quiet and private, ideally a bedroom. Cover a bed, or an area of floor if there is no bed, with a waterproof sheet and a blanket or towel. Ask the mother to empty her bladder into a receptacle other than a lavatory. She should then remove all the clothes below her waist and lie down comfortably on her side or on her back. Encourage her to relax between contractions and record their length and frequency. The cervix opens and the waters (amniotic fluid) may appear at this stage.

To assist the birth, you will need:
1. Blanket to wrap the baby.
2. Several towels.
3. Paper tissues, sanitary towels or clean cloths to be used as swabs.
4. Scissors and three 12-inch (30cm) pieces of string to tie the umbilical cord.
5. A saucepan or kettle of boiling water in which to sterilize string and scissors.
6. Clean water and soap to wash your own hands.
7. Antiseptic liquid.

Cleanliness is of utmost importance for the health of the baby and of the mother. Infection from your hands or from any of the accessories may prove fatal. Boil scissors and string for ten minutes, leaving them in the water until required, and wash your hands under running water for the same length of time.

The mother will feel the need to push down just before delivery. Rest between contractions is important at this stage. The mother should lie on her back and spread her legs apart as the contractions become stronger so that the first signs of the delivery can be seen.

When the baby's head is visible, rinse your hands in antiseptic liquid and cup them gently around the head. Do not pull on the head. As the head emerges ask the mother to stop pushing and to pant. This prevents the head from emerging too fast. Contractions may stop for a few minutes and the baby's head may rotate. Do nothing except support the baby's head.

When the shoulders appear, grasp the baby beneath the armpits and lift it up and onto the mother's abdomen. A newborn baby is slippery, so hold it firmly.

When the baby is completely delivered place it on the mother's abdomen with the head downwards to allow any mucus to drain from the mouth and nose. The baby's gasps and cries at this stage are normal and are the start of regular breathing. Wrap the baby in a blanket or towel and let the mother hold her child as soon as possible.

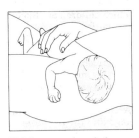

Holding a new born baby.

Wait for the placenta (afterbirth) to be delivered. This appears as a mass of red fleshy tissue and is usually delivered within about 20 minutes after the birth of the baby.

Tie the umbilical cord with a piece of string about six inches (15cm) from the baby's navel. Do not cut the cord unless you are sure that no medical help will arrive. If the cord must be cut, tie two more pieces of string tightly round it, one either side of the first piece. With sterilized scissors, cut between the two farthest pieces.

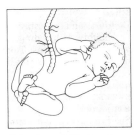

Tying the umbilical cord.

Complications

If the baby is born with the cord around the neck, loosen the cord and gently ease it over the baby's head.

If membranes cover the baby's face, they should be torn to allow breathing. If the baby does not breathe after delivery, give mouth-to-mouth resuscitation (see p.9).

If the baby's bottom or foot appears first instead of the head (breech delivery), do not interfere. Allow the birth to proceed normally, supporting the baby as required.

If contractions continue after the delivery of the baby and the placenta, a second baby may appear. The likelihood of twins is also indicated by the lump that remains in the abdomen after the first baby is born.

Bleeding after the birth may be due to part or all of the placenta being retained in the womb. Raise the foot of the bed and massage the mother's abdomen just below the navel. If the bleeding is heavy and does not stop within a few minutes, summon medical assistance urgently.

Emergency Treatment of Children

Many accidents occur to children as a result of their inexperience and natural curiosity. In most cases the injury itself should be treated as if it had occurred to an adult. This section is concerned with accidents and illnesses which children are likely to suffer and with the special precautions you must take when children are injured.

Remember, above all, that injured children need comfort and reassurance, that shock develops more rapidly and is more serious in children than in adults, and that in all cases an injured child should be taken to a doctor or a hospital as soon as possible.

Artificial respiration (mouth-to-mouth), heart massage and the treatment of choking
The adaptations of these techniques for the treatment of children are described in EMERGENCY FIRST AID on p.9, p.8 and p.13.

Asphyxiation
Remove the cause and give mouth-to-mouth artificial respiration. Do not blow too hard. See EMERGENCY FIRST AID, p.9.

Bites
Comfort and reassure the child. Rinse the wound thoroughly. If bleeding continues, press firmly on the wound until it stops. Take the child to a hospital or a doctor as soon as possible because antibiotic treatment, a tetanus injection and anti-rabies injections may be required. See EMERGENCY FIRST AID, p.10. For snakebite, see EMERGENCY FIRST AID, p.15.

Bruising
See *Fractures and bruising*, below.

Burns and scalds
If clothes are on fire, wrap the child in a blanket or anything that will smother the flames then cool with cold water or ice. (Do not use man-made fabrics such as nylon.) If the child is scalded, pour cold water over the injured area. Call an ambulance or take the child to hospital at once. Treat for severe shock. See EMERGENCY FIRST AID, p.10.

Children's illnesses
See under *Children's Problems* or under *Infectious Illnesses* in DISEASES, SYMPTOMS AND TREATMENTS.

Choking
See EMERGENCY FIRST AID, p.13.

Dehydration
This occurs more quickly in children than in adults and can develop even faster in babies. The symptoms are lethargy, a dry skin and a dry mouth. Dehydration may be caused by vomiting, diarrhoea or by sweating from fever or environmental heat such as too much sun. Frequent drinks of water, sweetened if possible, with a teaspoonful of salt in each pint of liquid will restore body fluid. If the child is vomiting, consult a doctor at once.

Fever and convulsions

In babies and young children, convulsions are often caused by a high fever. If convulsions occur, hold the child's head on one side and keep the air passage open so that the child can breathe. When convulsions stop, reduce the child's temperature by sponging the body with water. Call a doctor or take the child to a hospital immediately.

Fractures and bruising

For obvious fractures, see EMERGENCY FIRST AID, p.11. The injured part should be kept rigid with a splint or a sling and the child must be taken to a hospital as soon as possible. Bruising, pain, or lack of movement in a limb or sudden swelling in a joint may also indicate a fracture. If in doubt consult a doctor.

Nose-bleed

See FIRST AID TECHNIQUES p.32

Poisoning

See EMERGENCY FIRST AID, p.15, and see also FIRST AID TECHNIQUES, p.33.

Rash

In a child or a baby a rash may be a sign of over-heating, nappy-rash, an allergy to certain clothing materials, soaps, chemicals, foods, plants or drugs, or it may indicate such illnesses as chickenpox, German measles (rubella), measles or scarlet fever. Determine the cause and remove it if possible. Consult a doctor if you are in any doubt or if other factors, such as fever, are involved. Cover the area to prevent the child from scratching. A soothing lotion, such as calamine lotion, applied to the inflamed area may help to reduce the irritation.

Rescue from a height

The curiosity of an older child may lead to situations from which it is not easy to escape. Most commonly this occurs if the child climbs on a cliff or up a tree. When rescuing a child in such circumstances, it is most important to prevent panic. Do not show anxiety as this is likely to make the child anxious. Reassure the child and give advice about waiting in a comfortable position. Use a ladder to reach the child if possible. Otherwise call for skilled help, for example from the fire brigade or the coast guard. Keep talking calmly while waiting for help to arrive.

Travel sickness

This is common in children over the age of two and it tends to get better after puberty. It is a source of anxiety to the child and to the parents and the advice of a doctor is valuable. Anti-nausea (travel sickness) pills may help and may give the child confidence. Small plastic bags, with the means to close them, and a damp sponge should be carried when you travel.

Vomiting

Vomiting may cause *dehydration* in a baby or young child. See also FIRST AID TECHNIQUES, p.35.

19

First Aid Techniques

Abdominal pain

Mild pain may be relieved by resting and taking indigestion tablets. For severe pain, sit or lie in the most comfortable position. Pain in the lower abdomen is usually more serious than pain in the region of the stomach. If any severe pain continues for more than an hour, consult a doctor or go to hospital at once.

Allergic reaction

Mild allergies usually appear as local skin reactions to contact with plants or chemicals. Apply a cold wet flannel or other cloth to the affected area, but do not scratch or rub it. Call a doctor if swelling develops.

A mild face or body rash may also be caused by an adverse reaction to a food or drug that has been swallowed. Lie down quietly, but call a doctor if the rash gets worse.

Severe allergic reactions (anaphylaxis) are usually caused by drugs but may also be due to an insect bite or sting. In these cases a highly irritating rash covers the whole skin. The victim is also likely to suffer from breathlessness, collapse and shock. Place the victim in the recovery position (see p.12) and call a doctor, or take the victim to hospital immediately. Ask if the victim has any emergency medication such as an inhaler for asthma or antihistamine pills. If so, use as directed. Stay with the victim until help arrives. Observe pulse and breathing constantly as heart massage and artificial respiration (see pp.8-9) may be required. See also *Systemic and General Problems: Anaphylaxis* in DISEASES, SYMPTOMS AND TREATMENTS.

Asthmatic attacks

If the attack occurs indoors, the victim should sit on a chair with the arms braced on a table. This allows the chest and arm muscles to be used to help breathing. Try to keep the back straight. If outdoors the victim should use a fence, a gate, or the shoulders of a friend with the head resting on the arms. Tablets or spray may be found in the victim's pocket or bag, and the victim will know how to use them. If the symptoms do not improve after about five minutes call for a doctor or take the victim to hospital.

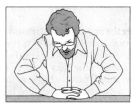

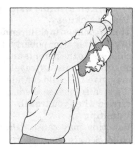

Asthmatic attacks may be relieved if the arms are braced to help breathing.

Back injuries

The casualty should lie face-up on a hard, flat surface, such as the floor. If the injury has been caused by a fall, do not move. Keep the casualty warm, by covering with blankets or a coat, and summon help. Call an ambulance if possible. Only if no help can be obtained should a person with a serious back injury be moved, and then only after the back has been completely immobilized with a long splint that stretches from above the head to below the bottom of the spine.

Bites

Animal and human bites (for example, of one child by another) should be treated as wounds. See *Bleeding,* below. First of all, the bleeding must be stopped, and the wound must be cleaned thoroughly. In the case of an attack by an animal, the animal should be investigated for rabies. As with all dirty wounds, immunization against tetanus may be required. See also *Insect bites and stings*, p.31, and *Snakebite*, p.33.

Bleeding — See also EMERGENCY FIRST AID, p.10

In all cases, bleeding must be stopped as quickly as possible. This is best accomplished by pressing on the wound. If the broken blood vessels are closed by the pressure and the flow ceases, the natural clotting agents can be effective. After bleeding has stopped, clean the wound thoroughly and take the casualty to hospital for immunization against tetanus. Anyone who has suffered major bleeding will also be suffering from shock.

For a small wound, firm pressure with the fingers is usually sufficient. A large wound in which many vessels are damaged may require a clean cloth to be held against the hole so that all the damaged veins are covered. A cloth is used for a large wound to allow pressure to be applied to a larger area, not to soak up the blood. For both small or large wounds, press on the wound as hard as possible for 20 minutes. Release the pressure after 20 minutes so that the rest of the circulation is not impaired. If the wound is still bleeding, press again for another 20 minutes.

Continuous bleeding from the mouth, ear, bladder or anus indicates an internal injury. Skilled medical treatment is required immediately. Lay the patient in the recovery position and call an ambulance. Only if no ambulance can be called should other means be used to take the casualty to hospital. Minor bleeding from any of these places also requires medical attention.

Breathing problems

Treat shortness of breath as an *asthmatic attack* (p.20). Rest, in a sitting position, improves the symptoms if the problem has nervous or emotional causes, but if breathlessness is severe or if it continues for more than 12 hours, consult a doctor. In an obvious emergency, call an ambulance or take the victim to hospital at once.

Bruising

Bruising

Bruising is due to bleeding into the tissues, which causes swelling and discoloration. It is usually caused by a physical injury, so make sure that there is no other damage, particularly to bones. If the swelling is accompanied by severe pain, take the casualty to hospital for further examination.

If there is no fracture, rest the area in an elevated position if possible or in a sling and apply a cold compress to reduce the swelling. Superficial bruises may also be caused by insect bites or by injections.

Burns — See also EMERGENCY FIRST AID, p.10

Burns caused by fires should be soaked immediately in cold water. If the fire is still burning or smouldering, the victim can be wrapped tightly in a blanket or coat, but not in anything made of synthetic material. Cold water is always best if available. Charred clothing will be sterile and should not be removed.

Chemical burns and scalds must be treated by soaking immediately in cold water, removing the contaminated clothing as soon as possible and washing the damaged skin thoroughly. Continue to soak with cold water for at least ten minutes, but do not rub the skin as this may cause further injury.

Cover the skin with a dry sterile dressing. Do not use lotions or ointments. Deep burns, burns caused by electricity and burns larger than half a square inch (a postage stamp) must be examined by a doctor as the true extent of the damage may be greater than it appears.

For large burns, call an ambulance as soon as possible because these are extremely dangerous.

Choking — See EMERGENCY FIRST AID, p.13

Convulsions

Do not disturb a person who is having convulsions. Move any dangerous objects, such as chairs, an electric fire, or glass, out of the way to prevent accidental injury. In a mild fit or in the case of a child with convulsions, gentle restraint may also help. When the convulsions are over, place in the recovery position. Call a doctor or send for an ambulance and stay with the person until the fit passes and consciousness is regained.

Cramp

An involuntary, painful muscle spasm that may affect the stomach or the extremities, particularly the legs and feet. The spasm is relieved by warming and massaging the affected part and often by stretching the muscles that are contracting. For example, to stretch the muscles of the thigh, calf or foot, try to straighten the leg with the toes raised and the heel pressed downwards. For cramp in the hand, pull the fingers firmly and steadily straight. Further cramps may be avoided by ensuring an adequate intake of fluids and salt. Consult a doctor if they persist.

22

Dehydration

This is indicated by thirst, lethargy and by the skin appearing to be dry and slack. It is likely to occur in hot weather or as a result of diarrhoea, vomiting and fever. It is particularly dangerous in babies and children.

Treat initially by giving fluids to drink, in small amounts, such as a glassful at a time. Add about a teaspoon each of salt and sugar to a pint of fluid. Too much fluid or fluid with too much salt in it may cause vomiting. If dehydration is associated with any other signs of illness, consult a doctor.

Diabetic emergencies

These are caused by an imbalance in the sugar levels in the blood. Either too much or too little sugar in the blood of a diabetic may lead to unconsciousness (coma).

Too much sugar, leading to a diabetic (hyperglycaemic) coma, causes symptoms that include thirst, confusion, fever, vomiting, deep breathing and the gradual onset of coma.

Too little sugar in the blood, leading to a hypoglycaemic coma, causes confusion, pallor and sweating. The coma develops rapidly.

If the victim is conscious, give some sugar, in the form of lumps or sweets, because a little more sugar will not harm a person with an excess of blood sugar whereas it will temporarily prevent a hypoglycaemic coma. In both cases, call a doctor or take the victim to hospital.

If the victim is unconscious, place in the recovery position and call an ambulance. Look for a medical identification card or disc round the victim's wrist or neck, in the pockets of the clothes or in any accompanying bags. Stay with the victim until help arrives.

Dislocations

Treat all dislocations as if they were fractures. Support the affected joint in a sling or on pillows. Send for an ambulance or take the casualty to hospital. Anyone with a dislocation is likely to be suffering from shock.

Drowning

Throw a life-belt or any other buoyant object to the drowning person. In general it is unwise to jump into the water to help another person unless you are a strong swimmer yourself. If you do jump in to help, remember to swim with a buoyant support to help the person float.

To resuscitate a drowned person, start mouth-to-mouth resuscitation as soon as possible. See EMERGENCY FIRST AID, p.9. Send someone else for help. Continue giving mouth-to-mouth artificial respiration until breathing starts again.

Ear injuries

If there is an object or an insect in the ear, do not try to remove it as the attempt may cause more serious injury. Take the person to hospital at once.

Electric Shock

Electric shock

Do not touch the victim. Switch off the appliance that has caused the shock. Check the switch, or pull the plug out. Use a wooden pole or a chair to move the source of the electric current away from the victim. Resuscitate the victim with heart massage and artificial respiration. See EMERGENCY FIRST AID, pp.8-9. When the victim is breathing normally, treat for shock. See EMERGENCY FIRST AID, p.13. Take the victim to hospital for treatment of electrical burns, which may be invisible on the surface but extensive underneath.

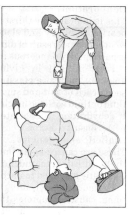

Electric shock. Switch off the electricity at the mains before touching the casualty.

Exposure — See *Hypothermia*, p.31

Eye injuries

A black eye is caused by bleeding around the eye socket. It may be caused by direct injury, or by an injury to another part of the head. To treat it, cover the eye with a cold wet towel for at least ten minutes after the injury.

Chemicals in the eye must be rinsed out at once. Hold the head on one side, with the injured eye on the lower side. Wash the eye with running water. Cover the eye with a clean cloth and take the casualty to hospital.

A foreign body in the eye must be removed as soon as possible without causing further damage. Roll the eyelid up by pulling on the lashes. Wash the foreign body out with water, or lift it out with the corner of a clean piece of material, such as a handkerchief. If there is continued discomfort, take the casualty to hospital.

Fainting — See *Unconsciousness*, p.35

Fish-hook injuries

Because a fish-hook is barbed it cannot be withdrawn through the place at which it entered the skin. It must be pushed round until the barbed end emerges, then this must be cut off. The hook without the barb can be withdrawn easily. Consult a doctor as a tetanus immunization may be required.

Foot injuries

These are most commonly associated with fractures. In such cases, and if there is no bleeding, leave the shoe in place to act as a splint. See *Fractures*, pp.26-27. If there is bleeding but no fracture, remove the shoe and sock or stocking carefully and treat for bleeding.

Fractures and bandaging

Any injury that may involve a broken bone or a dislocated joint should be treated as a fracture. Specific signs include pain that is made worse by movement, pain when the injury is pressed gently, swelling at the site of injury, and deformity of a joint or limb.

All fractures should be cleaned and covered if there is bleeding, supported with a sling or padded splint, and raised if possible to reduce swelling. The casualty should be treated for shock. Bandaging is the first aid treatment for many types of fracture and the techniques used are described on pp.26-29.

Splints must be rigid. They must also be long enough and wide enough to prevent any movement once the injured part is bound firmly to them. Padding is used so that the hardness of the splint does not cause further damage to the limb. A leg splint is illustrated on p.11.

If the collarbone is fractured, it is important to hold the casualty's shoulders back. To do this, tie a bandage round each shoulder by passing it under the armpit and tying it behind the shoulder. Use a third bandage to tie these two bandages firmly together, so that the shoulders are pulled backwards, and the broken ends of the collarbone prevented from damaging the lungs. Support the arm on the injured side in a sling.

If a rib is broken, support the arm on the injured side in a sling and take the casualty to hospital.

A crushed chest is particularly dangerous if there is a bubbling, gaping wound on the surface. Cover such a wound with a firm, clean bandage to prevent air from getting into the chest. Place the casualty in the recovery position, lying with the injured side of the chest next to the ground so that the sound lung can breathe more easily. Call an ambulance so that the casualty can be moved to hospital on a stretcher.

Fractures that affect the skull, face or jaw require specialized attention. Make sure that the airway is not blocked by the injury, and call an ambulance or take the casualty to hospital as soon as possible.

Spinal fractures are indicated by severe local pain over the spine, and possibly weakness, loss of sensation or paralysis of a limb or another part of the body. The casualty must not move or be moved because nerves or the spinal cord can be damaged. Call an ambulance if possible, and obtain the help of at least three other people. A stretcher is required: a large flat piece of wood, such as a door, will suit the purpose. Tie the casualty's legs together at the thighs, knees and ankles. Carefully lift the casualty onto the stretcher, preventing the body from moving, with one person holding the head, another the legs and the two others supporting the chest and pelvis. Tie the casualty onto the stretcher until you reach hospital.

Fractures and Bandaging

Bandaging is mainly used in the treatment of fractures. A bandage for support can be made from a belt, tie, scarf, or torn material. Most of the following illustrations show a bandage of the roll-type, which can either be bought as a roll or be made from a triangular piece of cloth.

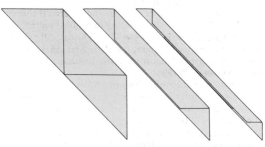

A triangular bandage can be made into a strip by folding the triangle from the point to the longest side, then folding it in half, lengthways, and then in half again.

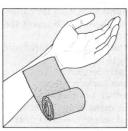

Start a bandage from the inside of a limb. Anchor the bandage with a double turn.

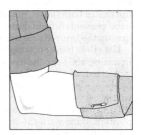

Finish a bandage on the outside of a limb, with the closure away from the body.

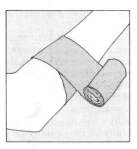

Wrap a bandage with the roll on the outside. Overlap by about half the width.

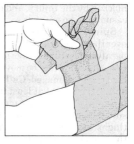

Unwrap a bandage by gathering the loose cloth neatly into the hands.

Fractures and Bandaging

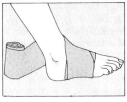

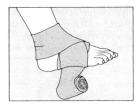

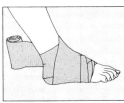

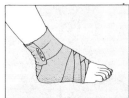

Foot and ankle bandages are anchored underneath the foot. The bandage continues in a figure-of-eight pattern around the ankle, overlapping successive turns so that the foot is covered to below the instep and the ankle is supported. For an ankle bandage, finish on the outside, as illustrated. For a foot bandage, continue to the base of the toes and finish on top of the instep.

Leg bandages start at the ankle and continue up the leg to the knee. Use a second bandage if the first is short.

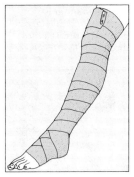

Varicose veins should be bandaged spirally to give support to the leg.

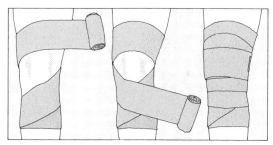

A knee bandage is anchored below the knee and bound in a figure-of-eight pattern that passes behind the joint, crosses the kneecap and finishes on the outside.

27

Fractures and Bandaging

Head injuries require bandaging if there is a wound that must be kept clean or if there is a dressing, for example one covering an eye or an ear, that must be held in place. A dressing should always be used with a head bandage.

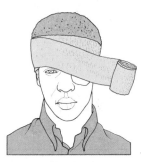

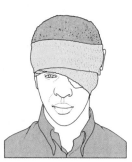

A head bandage is anchored round the largest part of the head. One turn drops lower than the others if *it is required to hold a dressing in place. Further turns make the bandage secure. It fastens at the side.*

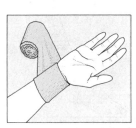

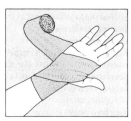

A wrist bandage is anchored round the wrist, then passed over the palm of the hand, in front of the *thumb, and round the back of the hand. This sequence is continued until the wrist is supported.*

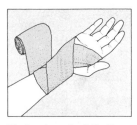

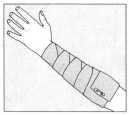

The bandage should be firm enough to prevent the wrist moving but should not affect the circulation to the fingers. *An arm bandage starts at the wrist and continues in a figure-of-eight pattern to just below the elbow.*

28

Fractures and Bandaging

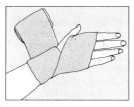

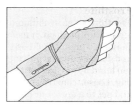

A hand bandage is anchored round the wrist, then passes over the back of the hand, across the palm

and back to the wrist. Subsequent turns cover part of the fingers. The bandage finishes at the wrist.

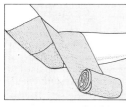

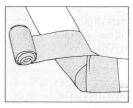

An elbow is made with a knee. The bandage is anchored round the forearm, then passed round the elbow

in a figure-of-eight pattern, crossing in front of the joint, finally finishing on the upper arm.

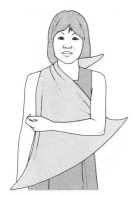

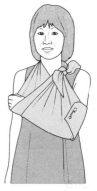

A sling is made with a triangular bandage. The longest edge passes over the uninjured shoulder, beneath

the injured arm, and tied at the injured shoulder. The injured arm is raised and the point pinned for support.

A sling is used to support an arm if the wrist or the fore-arm is injured or if the arm requires support following the fracture of a rib or collarbone.

Frostbite

Frostbite

Frostbite is skin damage caused by cold stopping the circulation of blood. It usually affects extremities such as the toes, fingers and nose. Do not rub the affected part, and do not warm by putting in hot water. Warm a frostbitten hand by placing it in the armpit, or get into a sleeping-bag. Loosen constricting clothing, drink something warm and get to a doctor or hospital as soon as possible.

Gunshot wounds

Gunshot injuries are characterized by small entry and large exit wounds. Treat as for severe bleeding. The victim suffers from shock and may also have serious internal injuries. Lay the victim on the floor in the recovery position and call both an ambulance and the police at once.

Hair round a finger

This is particularly likely to occur in babies and young children who twist their fingers in their hair. The tight hair constricts the blood flow and this causes the finger to swell. Hair removing cream or lotion must be used to dissolve the hair, before the finger becomes gangrenous. Visit a doctor or hospital as soon as possible.

Head injuries — See *Fractures and bandaging*, p.28

Heart attack

Check for the victim's pulse — see p.6. If this has stopped, give heart massage — see p.8. Mouth-to-mouth artificial respiration may also be required.

If the person suffers a heart attack but the heart does not stop, the attack should be treated as angina pectoris. The main symptom is central chest pain, which typically occurs as a result of excitement or exertion. The pain of angina usually spreads to the left arm and may also spread to the neck and abdomen.

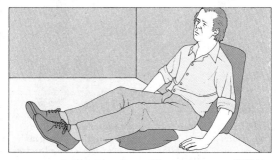

Heart attack. *If the heart is still beating the victim should sit in a comfortable position, ideally on the floor, with the back supported on pillows against a wall. This makes breathing as easy as possible. Stay with the victim until recovery is complete. Check the pulse regularly.*

Insect Bites and Stings

Heat exhaustion

Symptoms include extreme fatigue, dizziness, fainting, sweating and cramp. They are caused by excessive loss of salts and water in sweat, and may occur following exertion in hot, humid conditions. Give fluid to drink in regular, moderate quantities — one cup at a time. Add a teaspoon of salt to every pint of fluid drunk. Consult a doctor in case further treatment is required.

Heat stroke

The symptoms include collapse, a high temperature, a hot dry skin, and confusion, sometimes accompanied by loss of consciousness. Treat as for heat exhaustion, and move the victim to hospital as soon as possible.

Hernia (rupture)

Try to push the herniated bulge of tissue back into place and then consult a doctor. If the hernia is accompanied by local pain, swelling, general abdominal pain or vomiting, urgent medical attention is required as the hernia may cause an intestinal obstruction.

Hypothermia (exposure)

A condition in which the body temperature is dangerously low. It is particularly likely to occur in babies and the elderly in cold weather.

Wrap the victim in blankets or coats, and give warm, sweet liquids to drink. Do not give alcohol or use a hot water bottle or an electric blanket because these cause blood to flow suddenly to the cold extremities and so cool the body temperature overall, which may kill the patient. Consult a doctor as soon as possible.

Insect bites and stings — See also *Stings*, p.34

Medical attention is not usually required unless the reaction to the bite affects more than the local area of the injury, or the insect is poisonous. Treat a local bite with anti-irritant (antihistamine) cream or with cold water or an ice pack if nothing else is available.

Bees and ants have acidic venom, so apply a mild alkali such as sodium bicarbonate to the sting. The stings of wasps and hornets are alkaline, so a mild acid such as lemon or vinegar eases the pain.

Poisonous insects, such as certain spiders, scorpions and centipedes, are found in various parts of the world. If bitten or stung by one of these, kill the insect and take it with the victim as quickly as possible to the nearest hospital or poison control centre. Fatalities from insect poisoning are rare, but immediate treatment is always necessary. For the most effective first aid treatment of an insect bite, see the treatment of *Snakesbite*, p.33.

Ticks must be removed from the skin. Be careful not to leave the tick's head and jaws behind when its body is removed as this may lead to the bite becoming infected. Petroleum jelly, nail varnish, oil, alcohol or petrol may help to make the tick loosen its jaws.

Migraine

Migraine

As soon as the symptoms appear, drink three effervescent aspirin tablets in water. This form of aspirin is the most rapidly effective because other forms, even ordinary soluble aspirin, may be absorbed too slowly to have an effect. Lie down as soon as possible.

Miscarriage

Signs of an impending miscarriage include backache, abdominal cramps, and vaginal bleeding during pregnancy. If these symptoms occur, a doctor should be called at once. The woman should lie down on a bed covered with a plastic sheet and towels. The best position is on the back with the knees apart and slightly raised. Additional towels placed between her legs are also helpful. It is important to keep the blood that comes from the vagina for the doctor to examine. The fetus and afterbirth may not be noticed if the blood appears as a large clot. Examination of the fetus may indicate the reason for the miscarriage. When bleeding ceases, replace the towels with a sanitary towel, but do not use tampons.

Mouth injuries

An injury that causes swelling may block the throat and lead to suffocation. Stings and chemical burns are most likely to cause swelling. To treat these, the casualty should lie in the recovery position and rinse the mouth repeatedly with cold water. Sucking an ice cube also helps. Take the casualty to hospital as soon as possible. For cuts in the mouth, apply direct pressure on both sides of the tongue or cheek.

Nose-bleed

If the nose starts to bleed, sit with the head forward over a bowl so that the blood can drain from the nose. Breathe through the mouth. Press firmly on the soft lower sides of the nose to close the nostril for at least ten minutes. If this does not stop the nose-bleed, lie flat on the back. An ice pack held over the bridge of the nose also helps.

Old people with a nose-bleed may feel faint, and it may be better for an older person to lie down with the head supported by several pillows, rather than to sit with the head over a bowl. When bleeding has stopped, rest for a further half-hour and avoid sniffing hard or blowing the nose for 48 hours. If bleeding occurs several times, or if it continues for more than half an hour, call a doctor.

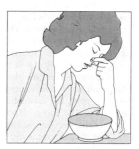

Nose-bleed. *Pinch the nose and lean over a bowl. Breathe through the mouth.*

Poisoning

In all cases of poisoning it is important to act fast. Call an ambulance and a doctor at once. In cases of gas poisoning, do not enter the room without proper breathing apparatus and skilled help.

If the person is unconscious, check for breathing (see p.6) and check for acid burns round the mouth. If the mouth is damaged and resuscitation is required, use the Holger Nielsen method (see p.14). Observe pulse and breathing until help arrives.

If the victim is conscious, ask the name of the poison. If strong acid or alkali has been swallowed, give the victim water or milk to drink to dilute the poison. Place in the recovery position and observe until help arrives.

If petrol or cleaning fluid has been swallowed, it is better not to induce vomiting as this may cause further damage to the mouth and throat. Place in the recovery position if the victim cannot walk.

For any other poisons, encourage vomiting by touching the back of the victim's throat with your fingers, by making the victim drink a pint of water containing two large spoons of salt, by giving a spoonful of ipecac syrup, or by giving more fluid to drink. Collect the vomit for analysis.

Always take a person who has been poisoned to hospital and always stay with the victim until help arrives. The hospital needs to know:

1. the name of the poison;
2. the time the poison was swallowed;
3. the time the patient was found;
4. whether the victim was conscious when found.

Also send any bottle or container near the victim, empty or half-full, and anything the victim has vomited.

Snakebite

Poisonous snakes are found in many countries of the world. The effects of their venoms vary from the mild poison of the adder or common viper found in most of the British Isles to the highly toxic venoms of the Indian krait, the African mamba or the American coral snake. Mild snake poisons may prove fatal in certain cases if the body reacts to them in an unusual manner. In such cases, shock or heart attack are likely to be the actual cause of death rather than the poison itself.

Identify the snake so that the correct antidote can be given. Kill it if possible and take it to hospital with the victim. In all cases, the first treatment of snakebite must be to immobilize the bitten part. Take the victim to the nearest hospital or poison control centre as quickly as possible for the appropriate antivenom to be administered. Do not use a tourniquet, do not cut the wound, and do not allow the victim to walk if the bite is on the leg. Reassure the victim and treat for shock.

Sprain

Sprain

An injury to the ligaments and tissues of a joint, commonly the ankle or the wrist. Initially the best treatment for a sprain is to apply an ice pack or a cold compress to reduce the swelling, then bandage following the directions given on pp.27 and 28. Rest the joint in a comfortable position. If in doubt, treat a sprain as a fracture.

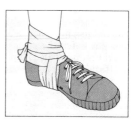

A sprained ankle can be supported temporarily by bandaging round the shoe.

Stab wounds

Do not move the weapon if it is still in place. Treat for bleeding, and stay with the victim, who will be suffering also from shock. Call an ambulance and the police immediately.

Stings —See also *Insect bites and stings,* p.31

Stings from plants or marine creatures such as jellyfish are painful and may cause extensive irritation of the skin.

Plants may irritate the skin by injecting a poison, or by secreting a fluid, usually an oil, that is absorbed by the skin. Symptoms include itching, followed by the development of a rash and sometimes of blisters. Wash the affected area thoroughly with soap and water to remove all the poison that has not yet been absorbed. Do not touch any other part of the body, especially the face or eyes. If any skin irritation causes more than a minor, localized reaction, consult a doctor.

Jellyfish stings are often painful and may be dangerous if the shock prevents a swimmer from swimming properly. Wash the inflamed area thoroughly with alcohol, with vinegar added to it if possible, but do not use fresh water. Anyone stung by a Portuguese man-of-war should be examined by a doctor in case complications develop. For other jellyfish stings, medical treatment is required only if there is an allergic reaction or if the patient suffers from a medical condition such as a weak heart.

Sunburn

For mild sunburn, in which the skin is sore and red but without blisters, keep the affected areas covered, wear a hat and use sunburn lotions or oils to prevent the skin from drying out. For severe sunburn, marked by pain and blistering, treat as a burn and do not expose the skin to sunlight until it is completely recovered. Symptoms of *heat exhaustion* may be associated with severe sunburn. To obtain a tan without burning, start sunbathing for short periods only, in the morning and evening but not in the middle of the day.

Zip-fastener Injuries

Toothache

If toothache is serious and persistent, a dentist or a doctor must be consulted. A throbbing, persistent toothache is usually caused by an infection such as a gumboil. Medical treatment is required but temporary relief may be obtained from pain-killing drugs such as aspirin, combined with a cold compress on the side of the face or drops of oil of cloves or alcohol applied directly to the painful tooth.

Unconsciousness

If a person is unconscious, check first of all for a fracture of the neck or head. If there is a fracture, do not move the casualty. If there is no fracture, check that the heart is beating and that the person is breathing. See EMERGENCY FIRST AID, pp.6-9. If the person is breathing and the heart is beating, determine the cause of unconsciousness if possible, and treat accordingly. Call a doctor or an ambulance, lay the casualty in the recovery position and observe pulse and breathing until help arrives. The following chart may also help:

If the person wakes normally:	1 Ask about possible reasons for unconsciousness. See also *Convulsions*.
	2 Ask the person to move limbs to check for injury or paralysis.
If the person is drowsy, but can answer simple questions:	1 Try to keep the person awake.
	2 Check for drug or alcohol abuse, poisoning or head injury.
	3 Look for identity bracelet or card indicating medical conditions such as diabetes or epilepsy.
	4 Call an ambulance or doctor.
If the person does not wake:	1 Place in recovery position and cover with a blanket.
	2 Call an ambulance or doctor.
	3 Observe breathing and pulse until help arrives.

Vomiting

Help the victim to sit, kneel or lean in a comfortable position, with a bowl or plastic bag within reach. A spare bowl or bag is necessary if vomiting is frequent or copious. After an attack, the mouth should be rinsed with cold water. If an attack lasts longer than two hours, call a doctor. Beware of the danger of *dehydration*, particularly in babies and children.

If there is blood in the vomit or if the vomit appears black and granular, bleeding in the stomach is indicated. Take the person to hospital as quickly as possible.

Zip-fastener injuries

These usually affect the skin of the penis, particularly of children. If the foreskin is caught in the teeth of a zip, it may be necessary to open the zip from the lower end by cutting the material in order to separate the teeth.

Survival Techniques

Basic requirements

Survival depends on an awareness of what may go wrong as much as on life-saving equipment. In the following pages, suggestions are offered which will help anyone caught unexpectedly in a dangerous environment. The kit is minimal and consists only of those things that can be kept in a car, in the bottom of a rucksack when walking in the wilds, in a locker of a boat, or in a cupboard in a weekend cottage. Although such a kit provides some necessary aids, the real secrets of survival are practicality, carefulness, and avoiding panic.

A basic survival kit should be simple and compact, and if it is made at home, the experience of making it will be useful if an emergency does actually occur. The kit should provide shelter, warmth, nourishment, and means of identification.

For shelter, a polythene sack, 6ft x 3ft (2m x 1m) is ideal. Alternatively a specially designed body-shaped bag can be bought. This must be windproof and waterproof. Use a piece of brightly coloured material that is easy to see. Anorak, rucksack, and the weatherproof bag can all be bought in bright colours such as orange or red. In a flat landscape, tie a piece of bright material to the top of a long stick or pole so that it can be used as a flag.

For warmth, carry matches, but not safety matches, and a piece of sandpaper in a sealed, waterproof container. Also carry some material that is easy to light, even when moist. A candle helps to conserve the supply of matches. Some types of cigarette lighter are designed for outdoor use and a lighter filled with petrol rather than with gas is preferable. Make sure this is filled before starting a journey.

For nourishment, carry food to last 24 hours. Include plenty of sugar, chocolate, nuts and raisins, and a few salt tablets. Even in a cold wet environment, carry a supply of water. Other highly condensed foods include stock cubes that can be mixed with a small quantity of water, condensed milk that is sold in a tube, and extra glucose or dextrose tablets.

For identification, use bright materials, a flashing mirror, a whistle and smoke from a fire to attract the attention of rescuers.

Additional items that are useful if there is space for them include a roll of coarse string, a rustproof knife, a torch, safety pins, a roll of strong adhesive tape, about 4yd (4m) of strong but fine gauge wire, a mirror made of steel but not glass, a loud whistle, and a reliable compass. If a magnetized piece of metal is used as a compass, remember to mark which end points north. Although these suggestions cover the most basic requirements, other things should be taken if possible. These are mentioned where appropriate in the following pages.

Survival in cold

The greatest danger to a walker or a climber who is caught in bad weather comes from hypothermia (exposure). This is particularly dangerous because cold and tiredness cause mental confusion which prevents the victim from noticing the early symptoms of exposure, such as slurred speech and lethargy, that precede unconsciousness, coma and death. It is of vital importance to recognize this lethargy and to oppose it by keeping active and awake. When these symptoms appear, the body needs warmth urgently. The person must drink warm liquids and be moved to safety at once. As a temporary measure, while waiting to be rescued, the body warmth of someone else may also help a person suffering from hypothermia.

Anyone planning to travel in cold conditions must take adequate clothing. In addition to the clothes that are worn, carry an extra sweater, a windproof garment that must be waterproof, a woollen hat, woollen gloves (preferably mittens) and a spare pair of long woollen socks. Wool is the best material, although some synthetic fabrics are also adequate. Cotton, even denim, offers no protection against wind and rain. All items of clothing must be large enough to cover the body. Shirts must be long enough to cover the small of the back and must also have long sleeves. Jackets, trousers and shoes must also be large enough so as not to restrict movement or the circulation of blood. Shoes must be waterproof, with strong, cleated, non-slip soles. Some protection for the eyes, such as dark glasses, is necessary in snowy conditions.

Survival in the cold depends first of all on keeping warm. The wind is the greatest threat, so find a place of shelter. Get into the large polythene sack from the emergency kit as soon as convenient. Shelter behind a wall if possible but avoid ditches or hollows that may fill with water. Use a plastic or nylon sheet to improvise a tent or shelter. If this is brightly coloured it will also help to attract rescuers. Use other emergency equipment to light a fire at night. Keep as dry as possible because dry clothes minimize heat loss.

If stranded by a snowfall, do not try to walk in the snow as the effort is particularly tiring. Keep warm by moving about in one place, but do not start to sweat. If you are covered by snow, whether in a natural shelter or in a car, make sure that you do not suffocate through lack of ventilation or because the roof of the shelter falls in. A stable shelter can be improvised by using slabs of frozen snow to build a thick wall and by roofing this with branches and more snow. When the snowfall ceases, leave a piece of brightly coloured material on the surface to attract rescuers, and do not let this be covered if snow falls again. Build a fire in a place that is sheltered from the wind. Eat small amounts of food regularly.

Survival Techniques

Surviving heat and drought

Body fluids are lost rapidly in hot conditions. Survival demands that this loss be minimized and, if possible, replaced. Water is much more important for survival in such conditions than food.

Preserve body fluids by keeping as much as possible of the skin covered. Despite the feeling of warmth, much less water is lost as sweat than if the skin is exposed. The head should also be covered. Avoid unnecessary exertion and if possible rest in the shade during the day and travel at night.

If no other water is available a small supply of drinkable water can be obtained by means of a simple solar still. This consists of a hollow in the ground that is completely covered by a stretched plastic sheet. Place a receptacle such as a cup or bowl in the hollow beneath the sheet and put a stone on top of the sheet directly above this bowl. Moisture is evaporated from the ground by the heat of the sun and condenses on the underside of the plastic sheet. The condensation droplets flow down to the point created by the weight of the stone and drip into the bowl directly below. Putting undrinkable fluid (such as seawater, radiator fluid or urine) or even green plants into the hollow increases the moisture of the air beneath the sheet and so increases the quantity of condensation and fresh water that is produced.

Survival in water

If you cannot swim, you should not go near streams, rivers, ponds, lakes or the sea without a life-jacket, because someone who cannot swim has little chance of survival in situations that are dangerous even for competent swimmers. The only way a non-swimmer can stay afloat without a life-belt or other form of support is to learn to lift the head above water, take a deep breath, close the eyes and float with the face under water until more air is required. Lift the head up, push down with the arms and take another deep breath. Do not try to keep the face above water all the time because this is too tiring.

This technique is also the best way a swimmer can keep afloat. Remember that clothes and shoes become heavy when waterlogged and should be removed. If there is a current, swim with it or across it, but not against it.

If you are in a boat that has capsized, hold on to it or to any part of it that floats, such as the oars. If you become tired, tie yourself to the floating object in case you fall asleep and lose hold. If the boat is floating properly but you are lost, keep the bows or stern pointing into the waves to prevent swamping. Collect rainwater in any available receptacle, including the sails, and use as little fresh water as possible. Never drink seawater. Improvise fishing tackle with string and bent wire.

Surviving in the wild

Some types of vegetation can be eaten but many are harmful if not actually poisonous. Any strange plant that might be edible should be tested by smell, appearance of sap, and initial taste. Plants with an unpleasant smell, a milky sap or a bitter taste should be avoided. If there is any doubt at all about the safety of eating a plant, stay hungry and avoid it.

Fish can be caught with a net made from a thin piece of clothing and a forked branch of a tree, and with practice a fish-hook and line can be improvised. Dawn and dusk are the best times for fishing, and fish can sometimes be attracted by a light.

Animal snares can be made from thin wire formed into a loop and tied to a tree or bush in a place where the animals are likely to pass. Learn to identify burrows and runs that are in regular use. Most fish and animal flesh can be eaten raw if necessary but meat spoils quickly and should not be kept.

Lightning

During a thunderstorm, the places that are most likely to be struck by lightning are solitary trees and tall objects. A person standing in the open, particularly on a skyline, is vulnerable and someone sheltering beneath an overhanging cliff or in the mouth of a cave is also in danger.

It is safest to shelter inside a building, deep in a cave or in a wood, but not against a tree trunk. If there is no shelter, lie down on flat ground or on the side of a slope.

Surviving a hold-up or hijack

Most important of all, appear calm and do as you are told. Do not answer back to anyone with a weapon, do not appear to disagree or criticize, avoid sudden or suspicious movements and keep your hands visible and your posture relaxed. Avoid eye-contact with the attacker, and do not talk to your companions unless you have been told you may do so. If shooting occurs, lie flat on the floor.

Escape

In general it is safer to remain where you are than to try to escape. This is as true for a hijack or hold-up as it is for a situation in which you are lost and alone. Only if you are in imminent danger or if there is no likelihood of being discovered should you move.

In the wild, it is important to wait in a place that is visible from the air. It is very dangerous to attempt to travel on foot in arctic conditions. In a desert or even in a hot climate such as jungle, it is better to travel at night and to spend the daylight hours resting. When resting in the shade, leave some visible signal in the open nearby to attract rescuers.

Survival Techniques

General advice

Always carry a map and compass when travelling away from civilization. Before you set off, make sure that someone knows the route you intend to follow and the alternative or escape route you will use if something goes wrong. Do not stray from these routes. When travelling in open country, always travel in the same direction. A compass or the stars can be used to help you keep a straight course. Follow water downstream, but don't get too close to the bank. When unsure of your way, mark trees or other objects you pass so that you can retrace your steps if necessary, and remember that it is unwise to travel too far each day, not only because this may make you too tired for the next day but also because you will need time and energy each evening to make a shelter, find food and light a fire.

First aid

You should always carry a basic first aid kit that contains, as a minumum, two triangular bandages, several big pieces of sticking plaster, antiseptic cream and several sterile gauze pads. A wide roll of sticking plaster is an alternative, but if this is carried, scissors are also required. A small container of antibiotic powder is useful to prevent wounds becoming septic, especially if you are likely to be away from base for more than 24 hours. A dozen medium-sized safety pins are necessary for securing bandages and for repairing torn clothing.

Signals for help

A fire can be used to produce smoke by day and a source of illumination at night. Be very careful if using this method in woodland. Collect both dry wood and damp leaves so that the former can be added to the fire at night and the latter during the day. On open ground, three fires in a triangle form an international rescue sign.

It is also possible to write on open ground. The letters SOS can be formed with stones or any material that stands out against the ground beneath. In soft ground, the letters can be dug in the form of trenches.

A flag on a long pole is useful in open country or on the sea because it is likely to be more visible at a distance than the person waving it.

If other people are nearby but appear not to have seen you, their attention can be attracted by whistling or shouting, or by flashing a light. Six even blasts on a whistle over the space of a minute followed by a minute of silence is an international rescue sign. Flashing a light is the best way to attract an aircraft or a ship. In order to direct a beam of reflected sunlight, hold the mirror in front of your face, point your finger at the person you wish to attract and tilt the mirror so that the sunlight hits your extended fingertip.

Systems and Parts of the Body

Introduction

An understanding of medical disorders and problems, with their symptoms and the ways they are treated, is based on a knowledge of the human body. The systems and various parts of the body are described on the following pages. A complete figure is outlined in each case to show how the system relates to the body as a whole, and the part of the body being described is illustrated separately to show its chief anatomical features.

Muscles, bones and joints are the mechanical structures that give the body its shape and enable it to move. Muscles attach to bones through ligaments and tendons. The forces exerted on bones by the action of muscles cause the bones to move against each other. Joints are the junctions between bones. The joints must be flexible and must have smooth surfaces to prevent friction, yet must be strong enough to prevent the bones from moving the wrong way. See pp.42-43

The nervous system and the senses control the mechanical functions of the body. The brain collects, coordinates, stores and recalls information brought to it by the sensory nerves from receptors such as the eyes, ears, nose and tongue. See pp.44-45

The heart, circulation and respiration work together to provide the body with oxygenated blood and to remove waste products such as carbon dioxide from the tissues. Blood is oxygenated in the lungs and is pumped round the body by the heart. The tissues absorb the oxygen and other nourishment (from digestion) that they need from the blood. See pp.46-47

The digestive system breaks down and absorbs as much as possible of everything that is swallowed. The waste is excreted as faeces. Cells lining the digestive tract convert substances into a form that can be transported by the blood to the liver and to other tissues where further metabolism takes place. See p.48

The urinary system includes the two kidneys that filter the blood, remove unwanted waste products of metabolism and regulate the balance of salts and water in the body. Waste products are stored temporarily in the bladder and excreted as urine. See p.49

The reproductive and endocrine systems are concerned respectively with reproduction and with the production of chemical messengers (hormones). The reproductive systems consist of the internal and external genitalia that produce sperm, in the male, and eggs (ova), in the female, and provide the conditions in which these can combine and develop. The endocrine glands produce the hormones that control metabolism and regulate the balance of fluids and salts in the blood. Hormones also control development and sexual activity. See p.50

Muscles, Bones and Joints

The diagrams on this spread illustrate the principal muscles and bones of the body and the structure of a joint, a bone and a muscle.

The knee joint, from behind, illustrates the relationship between bone and cartilage, and shows how ligaments attach to bone and bind the bones together.

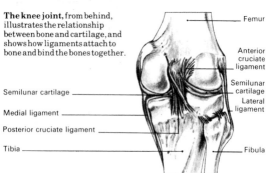

- Femur
- Anterior cruciate ligament
- Semilunar cartilage
- Lateral ligament
- Fibula
- Semilunar cartilage
- Medial ligament
- Posterior cruciate ligament
- Tibia

Muscles and bones of the body

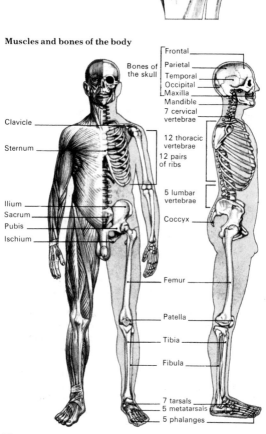

- Bones of the skull
  - Frontal
  - Parietal
  - Temporal
  - Occipital
  - Maxilla
  - Mandible
- Clavicle
- Sternum
- Ilium
- Sacrum
- Pubis
- Ischium
- 7 cervical vertebrae
- 12 thoracic vertebrae
- 12 pairs of ribs
- 5 lumbar vertebrae
- Coccyx
- Femur
- Patella
- Tibia
- Fibula
- 7 tarsals
- 5 metatarsals
- 5 phalanges

42

Long bones, such as the femur, are tubes with sponge-like centres filled with marrow at the ends. Blood is formed by marrow, mainly in the flat bones.

Skeletal muscle is under voluntary control. It consists of elongated cells that contract and relax rapidly, when stimulated by motor nerves.

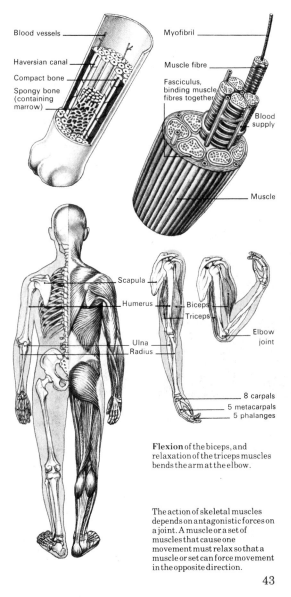

Blood vessels

Haversian canal

Compact bone

Spongy bone (containing marrow)

Myofibril

Muscle fibre

Fasciculus, binding muscle fibres together

Blood supply

Muscle

Scapula

Humerus

Biceps

Triceps

Elbow joint

Ulna

Radius

8 carpals

5 metacarpals

5 phalanges

Flexion of the biceps, and relaxation of the triceps muscles bends the arm at the elbow.

The action of skeletal muscles depends on antagonistic forces on a joint. A muscle or a set of muscles that cause one movement must relax so that a muscle or set can force movement in the opposite direction.

43

Nervous System

The nervous system is regulated by the brain, which receives and sends out messages through the peripheral nerves by way of nerve fibres in the spinal cord.

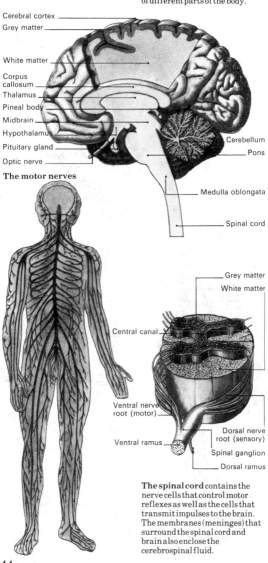

Areas of the brain record and direct sensations and functions of different parts of the body.

Cerebral cortex

Grey matter

White matter

Corpus callosum

Thalamus

Pineal body

Midbrain

Hypothalamus

Pituitary gland

Optic nerve

Cerebellum

Pons

Medulla oblongata

Spinal cord

The motor nerves

Grey matter

White matter

Central canal

Ventral nerve root (motor)

Ventral ramus

Dorsal nerve root (sensory)

Spinal ganglion

Dorsal ramus

The spinal cord contains the nerve cells that control motor reflexes as well as the cells that transmit impulses to the brain. The membranes (meninges) that surround the spinal cord and brain also enclose the cerebrospinal fluid.

The Senses

Sight, hearing, balance, smell and taste senses are each located in specific organs. Senses of touch, pain, temperature and muscular position are in the skin and muscles.

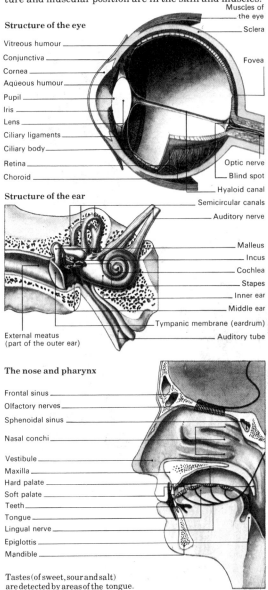

Structure of the eye

Muscles of the eye
Sclera
Vitreous humour
Conjunctiva
Fovea
Cornea
Aqueous humour
Pupil
Iris
Lens
Ciliary ligaments
Ciliary body
Retina
Optic nerve
Choroid
Blind spot
Hyaloid canal

Structure of the ear

Semicircular canals
Auditory nerve
Malleus
Incus
Cochlea
Stapes
Inner ear
Middle ear
Tympanic membrane (eardrum)
External meatus (part of the outer ear)
Auditory tube

The nose and pharynx

Frontal sinus
Olfactory nerves
Sphenoidal sinus
Nasal conchi
Vestibule
Maxilla
Hard palate
Soft palate
Teeth
Tongue
Lingual nerve
Epiglottis
Mandible

Tastes (of sweet, sour and salt) are detected by areas of the tongue.

Heart and Circulation

The circulating blood supplies the tissues of the body with nutrition (oxygen and food) and removes waste products such as carbon dioxide and urea.

The heart takes venous blood from the right atrium into the right ventricle, then pumps it to the lungs. Oxygenated blood returns through the left atrium to the left ventricle from which it is pumped through the aorta to the circulatory system.

Left brachiocephalic vein
Brachiocephalic artery
Left common carotid artery
Left sub-clavian artery
Aortic arch
Left pulmonary artery
Left pulmonary veins
Left atrium
Aortic valve
Left ventricle
Descending aorta

Right subclavian vein
Right pulmonary veins
Right pulmonary artery
Right brachiocephalic vein
Superior vena cava
Right atrium
Right ventricle
Inferior vena cava

Arteriole
Lymph vessel
Capillaries
Valve in a vein
Venule
Artery
Lymph node
Vein

Blood circulates through arteries which branch to form arterioles and then capillaries, where blood loses its oxygen to the tissues. Deoxygenated (venous) blood returns through venules and veins to the heart.

The lymphatic system drains the extracellular fluid and intestinal fat. Lymph nodes destroy invading bacteria.

46

Respiration

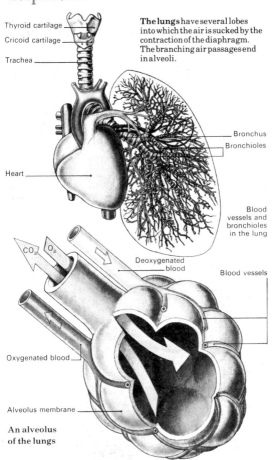

Thyroid cartilage
Cricoid cartilage
Trachea

The lungs have several lobes into which the air is sucked by the contraction of the diaphragm. The branching air passages end in alveoli.

Heart

Bronchus
Bronchioles

Blood vessels and bronchioles in the lung

CO_2 O_2

Deoxygenated blood

Blood vessels

Oxygenated blood

Alveolus membrane

An alveolus of the lungs

Blood-gas exchange occurs in the alveoli of the lungs. Capillaries that surround an alveolus carry blood containing carbon dioxide. Oxygen inside the alveolus passes through the surface membrane and combines with haemoglobin in the red blood cells. Carbon dioxide is released in exchange. Freshly oxygenated blood returns to the heart, and the air that is expired from the lungs carries the waste carbon dioxide with it. Cells lining the bronchioles and bronchi have hairs (cilia) that remove dust and mucus from the lungs.

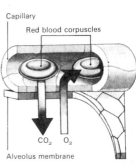

Capillary
Red blood corpuscles

CO_2 O_2

Alveolus membrane

Digestive System

Food entering the stomach may remain there for up to four hours. It usually takes about a day to pass through the digestive system as a whole.

Absorption of food occurs mainly in the narrow part of the intestine. This is filled with many small finger-like structures (villi) that give a large internal surface area lined with cells that absorb the products of digestion and transfer them into the bloodstream.

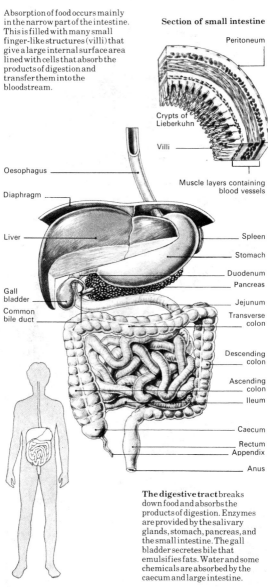

Section of small intestine

- Peritoneum
- Crypts of Lieberkuhn
- Villi
- Muscle layers containing blood vessels

- Oesophagus
- Diaphragm
- Liver
- Gall bladder
- Common bile duct
- Spleen
- Stomach
- Duodenum
- Pancreas
- Jejunum
- Transverse colon
- Descending colon
- Ascending colon
- Ileum
- Caecum
- Rectum
- Appendix
- Anus

The digestive tract breaks down food and absorbs the products of digestion. Enzymes are provided by the salivary glands, stomach, pancreas, and the small intestine. The gall bladder secretes bile that emulsifies fats. Water and some chemicals are absorbed by the caecum and large intestine.

Urinary System

Blood is filtered through the kidneys, and excess fluid containing waste products and salts in solution (urine) collects in the bladder.

Filtration occurs as fluids and waste products pass from a glomerulus of blood capillaries in the Bowman's capsule to the renal tubule (nephron).
Before the nephron drains into the renal pelvis, reabsorption of water and salts from the nephron concentrates the urine which is then collected and stored in the bladder.

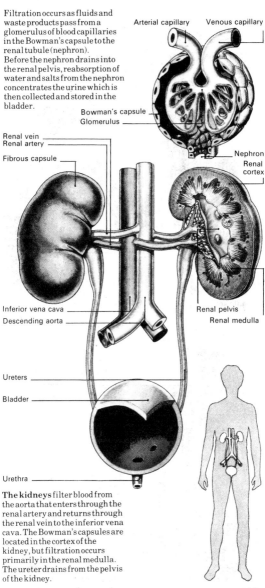

Arterial capillary

Venous capillary

Bowman's capsule
Glomerulus

Nephron
Renal cortex

Renal vein
Renal artery
Fibrous capsule

Inferior vena cava
Descending aorta

Renal pelvis
Renal medulla

Ureters
Bladder

Urethra

The kidneys filter blood from the aorta that enters through the renal artery and returns through the renal vein to the inferior vena cava. The Bowman's capsules are located in the cortex of the kidney, but filtration occurs primarily in the renal medulla. The ureter drains from the pelvis of the kidney.

Reproductive and Endocrine Systems

The main parts of the reproductive organs are illustrated.
Female organs are internal, whereas male organs lie both
inside and outside the pelvis.

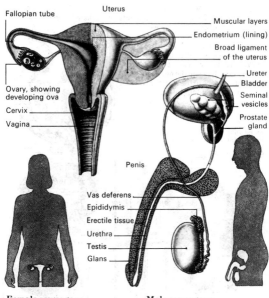

Female sex organs   Male sex organs

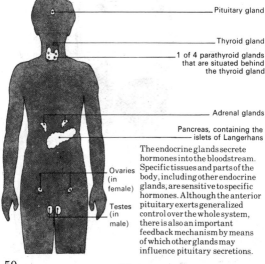

The endocrine glands secrete
hormones into the bloodstream.
Specific tissues and parts of the
body, including other endocrine
glands, are sensitive to specific
hormones. Although the anterior
pituitary exerts generalized
control over the whole system,
there is also an important
feedback mechanism by means
of which other glands may
influence pituitary secretions.

Medical Terminology

At a first glance, the jargon of a science may seem to be the hardest part of the subject to understand. In medicine, however, most terms are constructed from elements that have simple meanings, usually derived from words in Greek or Latin. The following list gives the basic meaning of some of these elements and illustrates their use with an example.

Element	Meaning	Example
a, an	without	*an*uria: without passing urine
ab, apo	away from	*ab*normal: other than normal
ad	towards	*ad*renal: towards the kidney
aden-i-o	gland	*aden*iform: gland-shaped
aesthe	sensation	an*aesthe*sia: without feeling
alg-e-ia-y	pain	an*alg*esia: without pain
andro	male	*andro*cyte: male (sex) cell
angi-o	vessel	*angi*ogram: X-ray of a blood vessel
ant-i	against	*ant*iseptic: against bacterial decay
ante	before	*ante*natal: before birth
arteri-o	artery	*arteri*osclerosis: hardening of an artery
arthr-o	joint	*arthr*itis: inflammation of a joint
auto	self	*auto*hypnosis: self-induced hypnosis
bili	bile	*bili*ary: of the bile
blephar-o	eyelid	*blephar*itis: eyelid inflammation
brachi-o	arm	*brachi*al: of the arm
brady	slow	*brady*cardia: slow heart beat
bronch-i-o	bronchus	*bronch*ospasm: spasm of bronchial tubes in the lungs
carcin-o	cancer	*carcin*ogenic: cancer-producing
cardi-o	heart	*cardi*ology: study of the heart
cata, cath	down	*cata*rrh: flowing down of mucus
cephal-o	head	*cephal*ometry: head measurement
cerebr-o	brain	*cerebr*al: of the brain
cervic-o	neck	*cervix*: the neck of the womb
chol-e-ia-o	bile; gall	*chol*ecystitis: gall bladder inflammation
chondr-ia-o	cartilage	*chondr*ocyte: cartilage cell
coel-e-i-o	abdomen	*coel*iac: abdominal
col-o-ono	colon	*col*ectomy: excision of the colon
cortic-o	outer layer	adreno*cortic*al: of the adrenal cortex
cost-o	rib	inter*cost*al: between the ribs
cox-o	hip	*cox*algia: pain in the hip
crani-o	skull	*crani*opathy: disease of the skull
cry-mo-o	cold	*cry*ogenic: temperature-lowering
crypt-o	hidden	*crypt*ogenic: of hidden origin
cut-a-i-icul	skin	*cut*aneous: of the skin
cyst-o	bladder	*cyst*ogram: X-ray of the bladder
cyt-e-o	cell	*cyt*otoxic: toxic to cells
dent-i-o	tooth	*dent*ition: arrangement of teeth
derm-ato-is-o	skin	*derm*atitis: inflammation of the skin
dipl-o	double	*dipl*opia: double vision
dips-o	thirst	*dips*omaniac: alcoholic
dors-a-i-o	back	*dors*iflexion: bending backwards
dys	abnormal	*dys*phagia: difficulty in swallowing
ec -to-tasia	outer	*ecto*derm: outer layer of skin
en-do-to	in; inside	*endo*crinal: secreting internally
enter-o	intestine	*enter*itis: intestinal inflammation
ep-i	outside	*epi*dermis: outermost layer of skin
erythr-o	red	*erythr*ocyte: red (blood) cell
ex	out	*ex*crete: evacuate
extra	outside	*extra*vascular: outside a vessel

Medical Terminology

Element	Meaning	Example
facient	making	aborti*facient*: making to abort
fibr-o-os	fibrous tissue	*fibr*oma: tumour composed of fibrous tissue
galact-o	milk	*galact*orrhoea: excessive flow of milk
gastr-o	stomach	*gastr*itis: inflammation of the stomach
ger-ia-o	old age	*ger*iatric: of old age
gloss-o	tongue	*gloss*al: of the tongue
glyc-o	sugar	*glyc*aemia: sugar in the blood
gnos-is-tic	knowing	dia*gnos*is: identification of a disease
gyn-ae-aeco	female	*gyn*aecology: study of female disorders
haem-a-at-o	blood	*haem*aturia: blood in the urine
hemi	half	*hemi*plegia: paralysis of half the body
hepat-o	liver	*hepat*itis: inflammation of the liver
heter-o	different	*heter*ogeneous: of different kind
homo-eo-o	same	*homo*genous: of the same origin
hyper	over	*hyper*active: overactive
hypn-o	sleep	*hypn*otic: inducing sleep
hypo	under	*hypo*thermia: lack of heat
hyster-o	womb	*hyster*ectomy: removal of the womb
iatr-o-y	medicine	*iatr*ogenic: caused by medicine
ile-o	of the ileum	*ile*itis: inflammation of the ileum (part of the intestine)
ili-o	of the ilium	*ili*ac: of the ilium (bone in the pelvic girdle)
infra	below	*infra*-axillary: below the armpit
intr-a-o	within	*intra*gastric: within the stomach
iso	equal	*iso*morphous: having the same form
itis	inflammation	*ir*itis: inflammation of the iris
kin-e-eto	movement	*kin*etogenic: causing movement
lab-i-io-r	lip	*lab*ial: of the lips
lact-i-o	milk	*lact*ation: the secretion of milk
lapse	fall	pro*lapse*: falling forward
leuco (leuko)	white	*leuco*cyte: white blood cell
lingu-a	tongue	sub*lingual*: under the tongue
lip-id-o	fat; fatty	*lip*aemia: fat in the blood
lith-ia-o	stone	nephro*lith*: kidney stone
ly-o-sis-so	dissolving	lipo*lysis*: dissolution of fat
lymph-o	lymph	*lymph*atic: of lymph or lymph vessels
malacia-o	softness	osteo*malacia*: softening of the bones
mamm-a-o	breast	*mamm*ary: of the breast
mast-o	breast	*mast*itis: inflammation of the breast
mega-lo-ly	great	*mega*locyte: enlarged red blood cell
men-o-s	monthly	dys*men*orrhoea: painful menstruation
metr-ia-o	womb	*metr*itis: inflammation of the womb
my-o	muscle	*myo*cardial: muscular cardiac tissue
myel-o	marrow	*myel*oma: tumour of bone marrow
narco-tico	numbness	*narco*tic: producing stupor
nas-a-o	nose	*nas*opharynx: nasal part of the pharynx
necro	death	*necro*phobia: fear of death
neo	new	*neo*natal: newly born
nephr-o	kidney	*nephr*itis: inflammation of the kidney
ocul-o	eye	*ocul*ist: eye specialist
onych-ia-o	nail	*onych*olysis: destruction of nail
oo, ovi, ovo	egg; ovum	*oo*cyte: egg cell
ophthalm-o	eye	*ophthalm*itis: inflammation of the eye
op-tic-to	eye	*op*tician: eye specialist
orth-o	straight	*orth*optics: straightening vision
os-se-teo	bone	*os*teometry: measurement of bones
ot-i-ico-o	ear	*ot*itis: inflammation of the ear
paed-ia-o	child	*paed*iatrician: children's doctor

Element	Meaning	Example
par-esis	weakness	myo*paresis*: muscle weakness
par-ous-a	bearing	multi*parous*: having many offspring
path-e-o-y	disease	*path*ology: study of disease
pector-i	chest	*pector*alis major: a muscle of the chest
penia	lack	leuco*penia*: lack of white blood cells
pep-sia-t	digestion	*pep*tic ulcer: stomach ulcer
peri	round	*peri*cellular: surrounding a cell
phall-o	penis	*phall*ic: shaped like a penis
pharmac-o	drugs	*pharmac*ology: study of drugs
pharyng	pharynx	*pharyng*itis: pharyngeal inflammation
phleb	vein	*phleb*itis: inflammation of a vein
phyla-c-ctic	protection	*prophyla*ctic: preventive treatment
pleur-o	rib; side	*pleur*odynia: pain between the ribs
poly	many	*poly*cellular: with many cells
pseud-o	false	*pseud*opregnancy: false pregnancy
psych-o	mind	*psych*ology: study of the mind
pulm-o-on	lung	*pulm*onary: of the lungs
py-o	pus	*py*ogenic: forming pus
ren-i-o	of the kidney	*ren*al calculus: kidney stone
rhin-o	nose	*rhin*itis: inflammation of the nose
rrhag-e-ia	outflow	haemo*rrhag*e: outflow of blood
rrhoea	outflow	dia*rrhoea*: outflow of faeces
rube	red	*rube*facient: making red
sarc-o	flesh	*sarc*oma: fleshy tumour
scler-a-o	hardening	*scler*oderma: hardening of the skin
seb-a-i-o	fatty secretion	*seb*orrhoea: excessive secretion of fatty substances
sect, section	cutting	hemi*section*: cutting into two parts
sep-sis-tic	decay	*sep*ticaemia: infection in the blood
sero	of serum	*sero*enzyme: enzyme in the blood serum
som-a-t-to	body	*som*atic: pertaining to the body
splen-o	spleen	*splen*ectomy: excision of the spleen
spondyl-o	vertebra	*spondyl*algia: pain in a vertebra
stea-to	fat	*stea*torrhoea: fat in the faeces
steno	contracted	*steno*sis: narrowing
steth-o	chest	*steth*oscope: instrument for examining the chest
sthen-ia-ic	strength	a*sthen*ia: loss of strength
stom-a-ato-y	mouth	*stom*atitis: mouth inflammation
syl, sym, syn	with	*syn*ergy: working together
tach-o-eo-y	fast	*tach*ycardia: fast heartbeat
tax-ia-y	co-ordination	a*tax*ia: lack of muscular co-ordination
tele	end; far off	*tele*neuron: nerve ending
therap	treatment	*therap*eutics: the science of healing
thorac-ic-o	of the chest	*thorac*otomy: cutting into the chest
thromb-o-us	blood-clot	*thromb*olytic: dissolving a blood clot
tomy	cutting	hysterec*tomy*: removal of the womb
ton-ia-ic	tension	myo*ton*ia: persistent muscle tension
tox-ic-ico	poison	*tox*aemia: blood-poisoning
trache-a-o	windpipe	*trache*otomy: windpipe surgery
troph-o-y	nutrition	a*troph*y: lack of growth
tympan-o	(ear) drum	*tympan*itis: eardrum inflammation
ultra	beyond	*ultra*sonic: beyond human hearing
ur-ino-o	urine	poly*ur*ia: frequent urination
uter-o	uterus	*uter*itis: uterine inflammation
vagin	vagina	*vagin*itis: vaginal inflammation
vas-i-o	vessel; sperm duct	*vas*oconstriction: narrowing of a blood-vessel
vesic-a-o-u	bladder	*vesic*ula: small bladder-like structure
vir-o	virus	*vir*ology: study of viruses
xer-o	dry	*xer*ostomia: dryness of the mouth

Diseases, Symptoms and Treatments

Introduction
This section is organized into 23 areas of medical interest, listed below, which correspond to various types of problem or disorder. A special section concerned with the problems of old age completes this part of the book.

The subjects covered by this section are listed alphabetically on pp.55-63. This index shows the group of medical problems in which the subject appears. If a subject, such as **Abscess**, appears in more than one subject group, all of these groups are listed.

The index also lists subjects that appear as part of another article. For example **Amenorrhoea** is described in the article on **Menstrual disorders** appearing in the major group called Gynaecological Problems. The index also includes entries that are described under an article of a different title. In such cases the index shows the group in which the subject can be found and the specific article in which it appears. For example, to read about **Allergic rhinitis**, look in the group called Nose Problems, under the article on **Hay fever.**

In the main text, a word printed in italics refers to the title of another article in the same subject group. For example, in the article on **Abdominal Pain** the word *appendicitis* appears in italics because there is an article on appendicitis in the same subject group (Abdominal and Digestive Problems).

Major Subject Groups

Index

A

B

Index

D

D and C, *see* Gynaecological Problems
Dead fingers, *see* Blood and Heart Problems
Deafness, *see* Ear Problems
Delirium, *see* Psychiatric Problems
Delirium tremens, *see* Psychiatric Problems
Depression, *see* Psychiatric Problems
Dermatitis, *see* Skin Problems
Development, breast, *see* Breast Problems
Diabetes, *see* Systemic and General Problems
Diaper rash, *see* Children's Problems: **Nappy rash**
Diaphragm (Dutch cap), *see* Urogenital Problems: **Contraception**
Diarrhoea, *see* Abdominal and Digestive Problems; Children's Problems
Diarrhoea, traveller's, *see* Abdominal and Digestive Problems: **Traveller's diarrhoea**
Dilatation and curettage, *see* Gynaecological Problems: **D and C**
Diphtheria, *see* Infectious Illnesses
Dislocation, *see* Joint and Bone Problems
Drug abuse, *see* Psychiatric Problems
Dysentery, *see* Infectious Illnesses
Dysmenorrhoea, *see* Gynaecological Problems: **Periods, painful**
Dyspepsia, *see* Abdominal and Digestive Problems: **Indigestion**

E

Earache, *see* Ear Problems
Ear discharging, *see* Ear Problems
Eczema, *see* Skin Problems
Emphysema, *see* Chest and Respiratory Problems
Enteric fever, *see* Infectious Illnesses: **Typhoid**
Epilepsy, *see* Nervous System Disorders
Epistaxis, *see* Nose Problems: **Nose-bleed**
Eyelids, *see* Eye Problems: **Lids, sore and swollen** and **Lids, twitching**

F

Fainting, *see* Blood and Heart Problems
False pains, *see* Gynaecological Problems
Fatigue, *see* Systemic and General Problems: **Malaise**
Fever, *see* Systemic and General Problems
Fibroid, *see* Gynaecological Problems
Fibrositis, *see* Muscle and Tendon Problems
Fingers, dead, *see* Blood and Heart Problems
Fissure-in-ano, *see* Anal Problems
Fistula, *see* Anal Problems
Fits, *see* Children's Problems: **Convulsions and fits**; Nervous System Disorders: **Convulsions and fits**
Flat foot, *see* Foot and Hand Problems
Flatulence, *see* Abdominal and Digestive Problems

Index

G

H

I

JK

L

Index

M

N

O

P

Pain, abdominal, *see* Abdominal and Digestive Problems: **Abdominal pain**
Paleness, *see* Blood and Heart Problems
Pallor, *see* Blood and Heart Problems: **Paleness**
Palpitations, *see* Blood and Heart Problems
Papanicolaou smear, *see* Gynaecological Problems: **Smear test**
Paralysis, *see* Nervous System Disorders
Paranoia, *see* Psychiatric Problems
Parkinson's disease, *see* Nervous System Disorders
Penis, discharge from, *see* Venereal Diseases
Periods, *see* Gynaecological Problems
Periods, painful, *see* Gynaecological Problems
Peritonitis, *see* Abdominal and Digestive Problems
Pertussis, *see* Infectious Illnesses: **Whooping cough**
Phlebitis, *see* Blood and Heart Problems
Physical problems (with sex), *see* Sex Problems and Sexuality
Piles, *see* Anal Problems: **Haemorrhoids**
Pill, the contraceptive, *see* Urogenital Problems: **Contraception**
Pink-eye, *see* Eye Problems: **Conjunctivitis**
Pleurisy, *see* Chest and Respiratory Problems
Pneumonia, *see* Chest and Respiratory Problems
Poker back, *see* Back Problems
Poliomyelitis, *see* Infectious Illnesses
Polyneuritis, *see* Nervous System Disorders
Pregnancy, *see* Gynaecological Problems
Pregnancy test, *see* Gynaecological Problems
Premenstrual tension, *see* Gynaecological Problems
Prolapse, *see* Anal Problems; Gynaecological Problems
Prostate problems, *see* Urogenital Problems
Psoriasis, *see* Skin Problems
Psychological problems (with sex), *see* Sex Problems and Sexuality
Psychosis, *see* Psychiatric Problems
Puberty, *see* Children's Problems
Pulse rate, *see* Blood and Heart Problems: **Palpitations**
Pyelonephritis, *see* Urogenital Problems

QR

Quickening, *see* Gynaecological Problems
Rabies, *see* Infectious Illnesses
Rachitis, *see* Joint and Bone Problems: **Rickets**
Rash, *see* Skin Problems
Rheumatic fever, *see* Systemic and General Problems
Rheumatism, *see* Muscle and Tendon Problems
Rheumatoid arthritis, *see* Joint and Bone Problems: **Arthritis**
Rickets, *see* Joint and Bone Problems
Ringworm, *see* Skin Problems: **Tinea**
Rubella, *see* Infectious Illnesses: **German measles**
Rubeola, *see* Infectious Illnesses: **Measles**
Rupture, *see* Abdominal and Digestive Problems

Index

S

T

Thrush, *see* Mouth and Throat Problems: **Moniliasis**; Urogenital Problems: **Moniliasis**
Thumb-sucking, *see* Children's Problems
Thyroid problems, *see* Systemic and General Problems
Tightness in the chest, *see* Chest and Respiratory Problems
Tinea, *see* Skin Problems
Toenail, ingrowing, *see* Foot and Hand Problems
Tonsillitis, *see* Mouth and Throat Problems
Toothache, *see* Mouth and Throat Problems
Tracheitis, *see* Chest and Respiratory Problems
Traveller's diarrhoea, *see* Abdominal and Digestive Problems
Tuberculosis, *see* Infectious Illnesses
Tumour, *see* Systemic and General Problems
Typhoid, *see* Infectious Illnesses
Typhus, *see* Infectious Illnesses

U

Ulcer, *see* Abdominal and Digestive Problems
Ulcer, mouth, *see* Mouth and Throat Problems
Urination, frequent, *see* Urogenital Problems
Urine, blood in, *see* Urogenital Problems
Urine, discoloration of, *see* Urogenital Problems
Urine, retention of, *see* Urogenital Problems
Urticaria, *see* Skin Problems: **Nettle-rash**

V

Vaginal discharge, *see* Gynaecological Problems
Vaginitis, *see* Gynaecological Problems
Varicella, *see* Infectious Illnesses: **Chickenpox**
Varicose veins, *see* Blood and Heart Problems
Variola, *see* Infectious Illnesses: **Smallpox**
Vasectomy, *see* Urogenital Problems: **Contraception**
Verrucas and warts, *see* Skin Problems
Vitamins, *see* Systemic and General Problems
Vomiting, *see* Abdominal and Digestive Problems; Children's Problems
Vulvitis, *see* Gynaecological Problems

WY

Warts, *see* Skin Problems: **Verrucas and warts**
Water on the knee, *see* Joint and Bone Problems
Wax, *see* Ear Problems
Whitlow, *see* Foot and Hand Problems
Whooping cough, *see* Infectious Illnesses
Wind, *see* Children's Problems
Worms, *see* Abdominal and Digestive Problems
Yellow fever, *see* Infectious Illnesses

When to Seek Medical Advice

A doctor should be consulted about all medical problems. In most cases a visit to a doctor or to a clinic for examination and advice is all that is required. More serious illnesses need to be reported to a doctor at once and emergencies need urgent medical attention. Such cases are indicated in the text by the following symbols:

H Call an ambulance or go to hospital immediately.

☎ Telephone a doctor for advice as soon as possible.

Anyone who is anxious about his or her health, for any reason, should always seek medical advice by visiting a doctor at the first convenient opportunity.

Abdominal and Digestive Problems

Abdominal pain. *Colic* in the lower abdomen may be severe enough to cause sweating and vomiting. Continuous pain, if accompanied by fever and abdominal tenderness, may be due to infection such as *appendicitis* or to gynaecological infection. If it is accompanied by backache and pain, with frequent urination, kidney infection may be suspected. A doctor must be called if it lasts more than four hours. If continuous abdominal pain is less severe, without fever, but is associated with nausea, *diarrhoea* or *vomiting*, it may be due to *gastric 'flu*. Recurrent pain may be caused by an *ulcer*. Pain from an ulcer is relieved by food, but it returns later as a dull, central abdominal ache. Conditions such as painful periods and *colitis* will also cause abdominal pain.

TREATMENT. Medicines for indigestion will often give some relief but a doctor should be consulted for the correct diagnosis and treatment.

Appendicitis. An acute infection of the appendix, a blind-ended finger-like branch of the large intestine in the lower right part of the abdomen. The cause of appendicitis is uncertain. The typical symptoms are abdominal pain around the navel which later shifts to the lower right abdomen, nausea, sometimes vomiting, and a slight fever, all of which develop over a few hours. The patient feels definite tenderness and pain when the abdomen is pressed.

TREATMENT. Consult a doctor immediately, and see also *Abdominal pain*. Surgical removal (appendicectomy) is usually required as soon as possible.

Colic. Colic describes the intermittent spasms of severe *abdominal pain* that may be due to intestinal obstruction, *gallbladder* or kidney disease, particularly stones in the kidney. Call a doctor if it lasts more than an hour.

Colitis. Colitis refers to two conditions, one mild and the other (ulcerative colitis) serious. The mild form is an inflammation of the large bowel (colon), producing intermittent *constipation* and *diarrhoea* and sometimes *colic*. The causes are uncertain. Ulcerative colitis is a severe illness associated with diarrhoea (often containing blood), fever and abdominal pain which rapidly leads to debility.

TREATMENT. Mild colitis is usually treated with anti-

Abdominal and Digestive Problems

diarrhoeal drugs and by increasing fibre and bulk in the diet. Ulcerative colitis usually requires hospital diagnosis and treatment with drugs and enemas. It is likely to recur and may require surgery to remove part or all of the colon.

Constipation. Constipation describes the inability to defecate because of hard faeces. It is usually caused by slight dehydration, by a lack of sufficient fibre and bulk in the diet, by failure to open bowels regularly when needed or by excessive use of laxatives. Rarely it may be due to a serious physical problem, and a sudden change in bowel habit should be discussed with a doctor.

TREATMENT. Eat a balanced diet that includes fresh fruit and small amounts of bran. Faecal softeners and lubricants may be helpful but avoid the regular use of purgatives. See also *Children's Problems: Constipation.*

Diarrhoea. The frequent passing of fluid faeces, which may be due to excess fruit, spices or rich food in the diet, too much alcohol, anxiety, *colitis, dysentery, gastric 'flu,* diverticulitis, *traveller's diarrhoea,* cholera, or to the excessive use of laxatives. Diarrhoea can be serious if accompanied by *vomiting* which will cause dehydration.

TREATMENT. Drink plenty of water. Use of a kaolin mixture or anti-diarrhoeal drugs may help. Before travelling abroad it is advisable to consult a doctor for a supply of drugs to control traveller's diarrhoea.

Flatulence. This is caused by an excessive amount of gas or air in the stomach or in the lower intestines. It may be caused by air swallowing, partial intestinal obstruction, gaseous drinks, some foods, *indigestion, gall-bladder disease,* or *hiatus hernia.* Anxiety may also cause flatulence.

TREATMENT. The cause must be diagnosed and a doctor should be consulted if the condition becomes severe. In minor cases, indigestion medicines and regular exercise for those who live sedentary lives will be helpful.

Food poisoning. This is indicated by an acute attack of *diarrhoea, vomiting* and stomach cramps, often affecting several people at the same time who have eaten the same infected food. It is usually caused by the toxins of staphylococcus bacteria, or of certain mushrooms or shellfish. In some cases organisms of the Salmonella group, which include the organisms causing typhoid and paratyphoid, infect cooked foods that have cooled. Botulism occurs sometimes but is rare.

Symptoms of the onset of staphylococcal, mushroom or shellfish food poisoning appear within an hour of two of eating the infected food and include stomach pain, acute diarrhoea and vomiting. The effect of Salmonella organisms that take time to grow on foods may not be felt for 12 to 24 hours but the symptoms tend to last longer. They are particularly severe in children and may be accompanied by fever, headache and general illness. Botulism is so severe and acute that immediate hospital treatment is necessary in order to save the life of the victim.

TREATMENT. An attack of food poisoning due to staphylococci or to toxins from mushrooms or shellfish is so abrupt that often it is over before a doctor arrives. The treatment is similar to that for *gastric 'flu.* A doctor must be consulted if diarrhoea and vomiting continue for more than 12 hours, particularly in children. Antibiotics are not usually prescribed as the

Abdominal and Digestive Problems

illness tends to improve naturally with the help of anti-diarrhoeal drugs once the stomach is free from the poison.

Gall-bladder disease. The gall-bladder lies under the liver. It excretes unwanted substances such as cholesterol and bilirubin in the bile. The gall-bladder also stores bile and discharges it into the small intestine where it aids the digestion of fat. Gall-stones, consisting of a sediment of cholesterol, bilirubin and bile salts, may occur in those with excess cholesterol in the blood or as a result of an infection of the gall-bladder (cholecystitis). Symptoms of gall-stones include severe *abdominal pain, colic,* sweating and *vomiting,* or possibly *jaundice* due to blockage of the bile ducts by a gall-stone. Chronic gall-bladder disease may be associated with colic or with no clear symptoms apart from darker urine and paler stools than normal.

TREATMENT. Appropriate antibiotics and admission to hospital are usually required to treat an acute attack of cholecystitis. Chronic infections will probably require an operation to remove the gall-bladder (cholecystectomy). About 20% of the population over the age of 60 have gall-stones. They need to be removed only if they cause symptoms.

Gastric 'flu. The term is used to describe the sudden onset of severe *vomiting* with or without *diarrhoea, abdominal pain* and *colic.* Typically it starts during the night and lasts 3 to 6 hours. This is followed by a few hours of extreme nausea, with occasional vomiting or diarrhoea before the onset of slight muscle aching, headache and sometimes a temperature of up to 100°F (37.8°C). The illness passes in 36 to 48 hours, leaving general malaise which lasts a further 2 days. It is caused by a virus infection (but not the influenza virus). The symptoms are similar to *food poisoning.*

TREATMENT. Do not attempt to drink anything until all vomiting has stopped, then start with sips of water and increase the quantity slowly. Ice cubes and mouth washes help. Call a doctor if the illness lasts more than 24 hours.

Heartburn. A moderately painful, burning sensation occurring behind the breastbone and in the pit of the stomach. This has nothing to do with heart disease but is a type of indigestion. It is caused by a spasm of the lower end of the gullet (oesophagus) aggravated by acid leaking back from the stomach. This may occur in *hiatus hernia,* after a large meal, when bending forward or after too much alcohol.

Hepatitis. A serious liver disease caused by a virus infection. Infectious hepatitis may be transmitted orally, by injecting with a dirty needle or through a wound. Serum hepatitis is caused by a virus transmitted by injection and particularly by transfusion of infected blood or plasma. The symptoms include weakness, fever, *nausea,* jaundice, and an enlarged liver.

TREATMENT. A doctor must be consulted and it may be necessary to admit the patient to hospital. Anyone suffering from hepatitis must be particularly careful with their diet and general health during the period of recovery, which may last for several weeks or months. Plenty of rest and a diet that avoids fats, fried foods, and alcohol, speed recovery. Careful personal hygiene avoids transmitting the disease to others.

Hiatus hernia. The diaphragm, between the chest and the abdomen, is weak at the point where the oesophagus passes

Abdominal and Digestive Problems

through it into the abdomen. Unusual abdominal pressure, due to pregnancy or to *obesity*, or a congenital weakness of the diaphragm, may cause a gap to develop in the muscle at this point. Symptoms include burping, hiccups, and *heartburn*, particularly when bending forward or lying down. The pain may resemble angina pectoris.

TREATMENT. Sleep propped up on several pillows. Frequent small meals minimize the effect of stomach acid secretions. Antacid drugs may also be helpful.

Indigestion (dyspepsia). This is a vague description for abdominal discomfort, stomach ache, *flatulence* or burping, sometimes accompanied by *nausea, heartburn* and occasionally *abdominal pain* in the pit of the stomach. Causes include anxiety, irregular meals, rich, large meals, and excessive smoking or drinking. It may be associated with *gall-bladder disease*, an *ulcer*, or *hiatus hernia*.

TREATMENT. Regular, light meals eaten slowly and avoidance of alcohol, rich spicy foods and aspirin-containing drugs are sensible precautions. It is also advisable to stop smoking, to get sufficient rest and to take regular exercise. Anti-indigestion medicines may help, but a doctor should be consulted if the symptoms persist despite these measures.

Intussusception. A bowel disorder in which the intestine squeezes its own internal surface as if it were a piece of food. The result is that part of the intestine is folded upon itself and this causes an obstruction. It is commonest in babies and young children. The symptoms include *vomiting* and *colic*, and sometimes anal bleeding.

TREATMENT. Urgent surgery is required.

Jaundice. Diseases that affect the normal excretion of yellow bile pigment (bilirubin) into the intestine, and so give a yellow colour to the skin and whites of the eyes, are known as jaundice. Specific causes include cirrhosis of the liver and forms of *hepatitis*, blockage of the bile duct (see *Gall-bladder disease*), and the excessive destruction of red blood cells found in haemolytic anaemia. Occasionally jaundice can be caused by other infectious illnesses or by drugs.

Liver disease. Many symptoms of mild ill-health are wrongly attributed to disorders of the liver. Despite this reputation, the liver is an organ of unusual efficiency and resilience, able to continue normal functions even when substantially diseased. Causes of liver disease include alcoholism, *gall-bladder disease, hepatitis* and some tropical diseases. Symptoms may be no more obvious than a vague malaise and loss of appetite, sometimes accompanied by *jaundice* and tenderness in the upper abdomen. Cirrhosis of the liver describes fibrous scarring of the internal structure of the liver. This may be caused by poisons such as alcohol or carbon tetrachloride, by nutritional deficiency or by disease.

Nausea. An unpleasant sensation of being about to vomit, often associated with abdominal discomfort, which may actually lead to *vomiting*. It may be caused by any disturbance or infection of the digestive system, by disturbance or disease of the organ of balance in the ear, as in travel sickness, by virus infections of the ear, by migraine, or as a side-effect of some drugs. Nausea may also be associated with pregnancy and with use of the contraceptive pill.

TREATMENT. This must be directed at the cause, but sips of

67

Abdominal and Digestive Problems

water, anti-indigestion medicines and anti-nausea drugs may help. A few long deep breaths may also alleviate the symptoms of acute nausea. Lie down if possible.

Obesity. The condition of being excessively overweight as a result of an imbalance between food intake and energy output. It may be due to thyroid problems or other endocrine disorders but it is usually caused by the habit of overeating which may be aggravated by depression and anxiety. It causes shortness of breath and may predispose the sufferer to skin problems, heart disease, arthritis, and diabetes.

TREATMENT. Consult your doctor for suitable dietary recommendations. Appetite-depressant drugs may be prescribed and hormone disorders treated if necessary.

Peritonitis. An infection of the membrane that lines the abdomen and surrounds the abdominal organs. Peritonitis may be caused by an infection or rupture of an abdominal structure. This may occur in *appendicitis*, salpingitis, diverticulitis, or as a result of a burst peptic *ulcer*. Symptoms include severe *abdominal pain*, fever, and often *vomiting*.

TREATMENT. Immediate admission to hospital is required for an operation to drain the infection, followed by skilled nursing care and antibiotic treatment.

Rupture (hernia). Rupture describes not only the breaking or tearing of tissue (as in a ruptured appendix in *appendicitis*) but also a hernia which is due to weakness in the muscles covering part of the abdomen. This weakness allows internal structures to push through the muscle wall. A hernia may occur in the groin (inguinal and femoral hernia), at the umbilicus (umbilical hernia), and occasionally elsewhere, for instance at the site of a scar or through the diaphragm (see *Hiatus hernia*).

TREATMENT. An operation is the only effective cure for a hernia, but a truss may be helpful as a temporary measure.

Stomach ache. A diffuse abdominal discomfort, seldom severe enough to cause pain or interfere with normal work. It is usually associated with *indigestion*. See also *Abdominal pain, Flatulence* and *Nausea*.

Traveller's diarrhoea. This is a general name for intestinal disorders that occur following a change in country, climate and diet. The usual causes are a change in diet, excessive intake of fruit, especially if this is not carefully washed, unusually large quantities of alcohol, particularly wine, inadequate sanitation, or true intestinal infections.

TREATMENT. Do not drink water that has not been boiled or sterilized. Drinking water can be bought in many countries. Take care with alcohol and dietary excess and avoid pre-cooked foods and unwashed and unpeeled fruit. Proprietary drugs, without a prescription, seldom help. During the attack itself, drink plenty of fluids, if necessary with extra salt, to prevent dehydration. Use anti-diarrhoeal medicines recommended by a doctor. If severe diarrhoea persists for more than 24 hours, particularly if associated with a fever or dehydration, consult a doctor.

Ulcer. A peptic ulcer occurs because excess acid erodes the wall of the stomach or the duodenum. Many factors may contribute to this damage, usually by affecting the normally protective lining of the stomach. An acute ulcer may be caused in this way by alcohol, aspirin, anti-rheumatic or corticosteroid drugs, or by acute stress resulting from an operation or from burns. Chronic ulcers occur more often in middle-aged men than women. Most affect the duodenum and are probably influenced by long-term stress, excessive alcohol consumption and smoking. Symptoms include attacks of upper *abdominal pain,* occurring about two hours after a meal and often accompanied by *heartburn, nausea* and *vomiting.* These may be relieved by milk and antacids.

TREATMENT. Medical treatment with antacids and drugs helps to reduce acid secretion as does a diet of small, regular, bland meals. Smoking and alcohol and foods that aggravate the stomach, such as spiced or fried foods, should all be avoided. Surgery is indicated if other treatment fails, if there is evidence of bleeding, if the ulcer perforates the stomach lining, or if extreme scarring causes obstruction.

Vomiting. Vomiting may be caused by *gastric 'flu, food poisoning, travel sickness, nausea,* infectious hepatitis, pregnancy, the use of oral contraceptives, gastrointestinal obstruction, dietary or alcohol excess, or an overdose of medically prescribed drugs. It may also be associated with anorexia nervosa, migraine or *abdominal pain* and *diarrhoea.*

TREATMENT. Treatment must be directed at the cause, but to take sips of water or to suck ice cubes and to lie down and keep warm all help. Consult a doctor if vomiting occurs as frequently as once or twice an hour for more than 4 hours, if it is associated with pain, or if it continues for more than a day. See also *Children's Problems: Vomiting.*

Worms. Parasitic worms are commonly transmitted by contaminated food or water or by the bites of certain animals or insects.

There are two main groups of parasitic worms. (1) The roundworms such as ascaris, enterobius (pinworm), and trichuris (whipworm) infest the intestine. The Filarioidea invade body tissues, causing filariasis. (2) The flatworms include flukes, which invade the body tissues to form cysts, and tapeworms, which usually inhabit the intestine.

TREATMENT. A diagnosis is usually made by finding worms in the faeces. They seldom cause intestinal pain or diarrhoea but may cause listlessness. A doctor may prescribe medication to kill the worms. Infection of the body tissues requires special investigation and treatment.

Anal Problems

Abscess. A region of infected tissue in the anus. It is caused by local infection which may be due to *fissure-in-ano,* tuberculosis or, occasionally, cancer. Symptoms include swelling and severely throbbing local pain made worse by defecation. Sometimes bleeding and discharge through a *fistula* occur.
TREATMENT. An operation is required, under general anaesthesia, to drain the abscess. Careful attention with antiseptic dressings usually leads to rapid healing.

Bleeding. The painless loss of bright red blood is usually due to *haemorrhoids* but may also be caused by diverticulitis, intussusception, an inflammatory disease such as ulcerative colitis, cancer or a benign *tumour.* Dark grey or black blood (melaena) usually comes from higher in the digestive tract, often from a stomach ulcer. Painful bleeding usually indicates an *abscess* or a *fistula.*

Anal Problems

TREATMENT. It is important to consult a doctor. A special instrument (a proctoscope or a sigmoidoscope) may be used to examine the intestine or the intestine may be studied by means of X-rays following a barium enema.

Fissure-in-ano. A crack in the skin of the anus which may occur after constipation. It is painful and often causes bleeding on defecation. It is not uncommon in babies and in the elderly.

TREATMENT. 1. Local anaesthetic ointments or suppositories applied before defecation. 2. Lubricants and roughage in the diet to produce large, soft stools. 3. Sometimes an operation is required to stretch the anal muscle.

Fistula. An abnormal channel between the internal surface of the anus and the surrounding skin. It is usually caused by recurrent abscess formation, sometimes associated with ulcerative colitis or tuberculosis. The symptoms include pain and the discharge of foul-smelling pus.

TREATMENT. An operation, under general anaesthetic, is required to open the channel.

Haemorrhoids (piles). Dilated veins that occur inside or outside the ring of anal muscle. They are caused by constipation, diarrhoea, pressure on local veins during pregnancy or, occasionally, by a tumour. Symptoms include bleeding, itching and soreness, with a protruding lump.

TREATMENT. 1. Washing and careful drying of the area twice a day and regular defecation. If necessary, mild laxatives may be used. Additional fibre bulk in the diet assists the treatment. 2. Ointments and suppositories may be used overnight. 3. Anaesthetic and antibiotic preparations are sometimes prescribed by a doctor. 4. Injections may also be given deliberately to cause thrombosis (blood-clotting) of the piles and scarring, which produces minor discomfort and is usually done in the surgery. 5. Anal muscle can be stretched under general anaesthetic. 6. Surgical removal of the piles (haemorrhoidectomy) is a more complicated operation and may require seven to ten days in hospital.

Itching. A sign of mild infection of the moist skin of the anus. It may be due to *haemorrhoids*, to a side-effect of antibiotic treatment or to infection with threadworms.

TREATMENT. Washing twice daily, careful drying and dusting with unscented talcum powder. Application of haemorrhoid cream may help, but if this fails consult a doctor.

Lump. This is almost always a *haemorrhoid* protruding from the anus, but it may also be due to an *abscess,* a polyp of the rectum or a *prolapse* of the mucosa (intestinal lining). In babies it may indicate a prolapse of the mucosa or an intussusception.

Prolapse. A relatively rare occurrence in which the mucosal lining of the rectum separates from the muscle wall and hangs out through the anus. This may occur spontaneously in infants. It may also be caused by haemorrhoids or recurrent constipation. It appears as a bulge of soft, red tissue hanging out of the anus.

TREATMENT. In infants it is self-curing. In adults the excess mucosa may be cut off in an operation and the edges joined together, or the patient may be given special injections which produce scarring and thereby cause the mucosa to adhere to the muscle wall. In certain cases a wire ring may be used to narrow the anal opening.

Back Problems

Backache. This can be due to muscle, ligament, bone or nerve injury or it may be caused by an ailment in an underlying part, such as the kidney. The sudden onset of backache is usually due to a torn muscle or ligament or, occasionally, to the fracture of part of a vertebra. Kidney infection (pyelitis) causes pain on one side with fever and frequent urination. Lung infections, such as pleurisy, cause pain in the back of the chest wall accompanied by fever and cough. Painful periods (dysmenorrhoea) cause low central backache.

TREATMENT. Minor muscle and ligament injuries usually settle in a few days with rest and care with movement. More severe pain requires a doctor's examination. Pain-killing and muscle-relaxing drugs and sometimes an injection of local anaesthetic often help. All such ailments require a doctor's diagnosis if they last for more than 24 hours.

Bent or curved back. If this occurs suddenly and is painful it is due to muscle spasm or spinal injury. See *Backache*. If onset is gradual, between the ages of 10 and 20, it needs specialist assessment and treatment. This is more common in girls and the cause is uncertain. If it occurs between the ages of 20 and 40 it is often due to bamboo spine (ankylosing spondylitis), which is a rheumatic condition causing deformity and stiffening of the spine, and requires specialist treatment. If it occurs after 40 years of age it is usually due to gradual loss of calcium from the vertebrae (osteoporosis) with gradual flattening of the bones leading to spinal deformity, the bent back of old age.

Hunchback. This may be a severe form of *bent or curved back* or it may be due to tuberculosis of the spine when a child, which causes the collapse of one or two vertebrae leading to the deformity.

TREATMENT. To be successful, treatment must begin as soon as the disorder starts to develop.

Lumbago. A term for low *backache* in the lumbar region.

Poker back. This is due to rigidity of the lower spine caused by the rheumatic condition ankylosing spondylitis. See also *Bent or curved back*.

Sciatica. Pressure on part of the sciatic nerve, which runs from the lower spine down the back of the thigh and leg to the foot, causes pain and, sometimes, numbness in the parts of the leg supplied by the nerve. Sciatica is usually caused by arthritis of the spine or a *slipped disc.*

TREATMENT. A definite diagnosis must be made by a doctor, if necessary with the aid of X-rays and blood tests. The doctor may prescribe pain-killing and anti-rheumatic drugs. Physiotherapy can teach correct bending with a straight back and bent knees and can strengthen back muscles.

Slipped disc. Each bone (vertebra) in the spine has a thick pad of fibrous tissue between it and the next one. This disc-shaped pad has a softer jelly-like centre. If the fibrous tissue tears, the softer centre can protrude to press on a nerve, and so cause pain and loss of sensation, as in *sciatica.*

TREATMENT. The protrusion eventually diminishes in size if the patient rests. Anti-rheumatic drugs may help this process. Manipulation or stretching the spine (traction) causes a change in direction of the protrusion and may relieve pressure on the nerve.

Blood and Heart Problems

Blood and Heart Problems

Anaemia. A reduction in the oxygen-carrying capacity of the blood. Symptoms are negligible in mild cases but in more severe cases paleness, breathlessness, *palpitations*, and fatigue may all occur.

TREATMENT. This depends on the cause but in most cases additional vitamins, iron and, rarely, corticosteroid drugs may be required. If anaemia is caused by severe bleeding from post-operative haemorrhage, from a wound, or from a bleeding stomach ulcer, rapid emergency treatment is required. In less severe cases, caused by recurrent nose-bleeds or heavy periods, the cause should be treated and iron tablets should be taken.

Inadequate production of oxygen-carrying red blood cells may be due to nutritional deficiencies of iron, vitamin B_{12} (the lack of which causes pernicious anaemia), folic acid, vitamin C or trace elements such as copper or cobalt.

Rapid destruction of red blood cells (haemolytic anaemia) may occur in malaria and in adverse reactions to some drugs. It may also occur when the red blood cells are unusually fragile from a congenital fault, as in sickle-cell anaemia and thalassaemia.

Angina pectoris. Angina pectoris is a pain in the chest caused by lack of oxygen reaching the heart muscle. It is usually brought on by exercise. Typical symptoms include a constricting pain in the centre of the chest which may spread to the neck and jaw, to the shoulders, and down one or both arms to the hand. It is sometimes accompanied by breathlessness, faintness or sweating. It disappears with rest.

TREATMENT. Specific drugs to relieve pain and to dilate blood vessels may be prescribed. Angina pectoris is often a sign of heart disease but it does not invariably lead to a *heart attack* and care with diet and exercise may do much to prevent the development of heart disease if it is present.

Arteriosclerosis (hardening of the arteries). This is reduced elasticity of an artery due to thickening of the artery wall. It is made worse by hypertension, by high levels of cholesterol and fatty substances in the blood, by smoking, or by diabetes. Initially no symptoms are evident but the patient is in danger of suffering *thrombosis, heart attack, stroke* or pain in the calves when walking.

TREATMENT. Prevention is easier than cure. Regular exercise to the point of slight shortness of breath, and a reduction of cholesterol levels in the blood by diet, are necessary. Stopping smoking, reducing weight, and, occasionally, arterial surgery to remove a segment of a damaged artery, are also important in the control of this disease.

Blood pressure. High blood pressure (hypertension) is usually associated with narrowing of the peripheral blood vessels, as in *arteriosclerosis,* or with hormone disorders or kidney diseases. Blood pressure may be lower than normal following an illness. Low blood pressure (hypotension) increases the likelihood of *fainting* caused by a reduction in the blood supply to the brain.

TREATMENT. As high blood pressure is often associated with obesity and anxiety these should be treated initially. Certain drugs reduce the pressure to normal but a doctor must decide whether treatment is required or not.

Blood and Heart Problems

Circulation problems. The body may be affected in a variety of ways because of problems with the circulation of blood. Abnormalities in the constriction or dilatation of peripheral vessels may develop with age and result in the *dead fingers* and cyanosis of the extremities found often in the elderly. Similarly, poor general circulation may also cause chilblains, and a diminished circulation to the brain will cause a person to faint. The blue baby syndrome is caused by inadequate oxygenation of the tissues, and this may be a circulatory or a respiratory problem. Diseases such as *arteriosclerosis, phlebitis* and *varicose veins* also affect the general circulation and so may increase the likelihood of a person suffering a deep venous *thrombosis,* a *stroke* or *heart failure.*
TREATMENT. Specific conditions require particular treatments. To help prevent circulation problems as you grow older, stop smoking, lose weight and eat a balanced diet, avoiding saturated (animal) fats and too many carbohydrates, and making sure of an adequate intake of vitamins and minerals. Take regular exercise that is strenuous enough to give shortness of breath.

Dead fingers. A sensation of numbness in the fingers often accompanied by stiffness. The cause is seldom serious unless there is a fracture of the elbow that obstructs the blood supply. An unusual sensitivity of the blood vessels to cold also causes numbness and paleness of the fingers.

Fainting (syncope). Fainting is caused by a sudden drop in blood pressure which reduces the supply of blood to the brain and so causes a temporary loss of consciousness. Fainting may be associated with fever, *anaemia,* pregnancy, fatigue, hunger, standing for a long time, some drugs or bleeding following an injury. Slight giddiness, dry mouth, cold sweat, difficulty in seeing clearly, and nausea may all precede a faint and give sufficient warning that one should lie down or put one's head between one's knees.

Gangrene. The death of an area of tissue that is still part of a living body. It is usually caused by blockage of the blood supply to the affected area. This may be the result of an accident, of severe *arteriosclerosis,* of infection, or possibly of frostbite. Dry gangrene usually affects the extremities, particularly the toes or fingers. The tissues are seen to shrivel and darken. Sudden blockage of an artery leads to painful swelling of the area, which may then become infected. Infection, particularly if the blood supply is poor, may lead to infective gangrene, with black, wet, discharging tissue.

Gas gangrene is a severe form of infection in the tissues as a result of a wound. It is associated with the production of gas and poisons by bacteria in the infected tissue that can ultimately affect the whole body and cause death.
TREATMENT. Consult a doctor at once. Cover the area with a light, dry dressing. Do not warm the area. Admission to hospital may be necessary for appropriate treatment with antibiotics and dressings to kill any infection. Sometimes an operation is required to improve the blood supply.

Heart attack. A lay term for a coronary thrombosis (myocardial infarction) caused by the blockage of a branch of a coronary artery. This blockage prevents oxygenated blood from reaching part of the heart muscle, and so affects the action of the heart. Typical symptoms include severe, constricting, mid-

Blood and Heart Problems

chest pain that may spread to one or both shoulders, down the arms to the hands, up the neck to the jaw and into the upper abdomen. This pain is often accompanied by nausea, vomiting and sweating and may be followed by shock, due to the drop in blood pressure, and irregular pulse.

TREATMENT. For heart massage, see FIRST AID, pp. 8-9. As the patient recovers from the heart attack bed rest at home or special nursing in a coronary-care unit in a hospital are required. Anticoagulant drugs may be given in certain cases. Following recovery the patient should take regular exercise, lose weight, stop smoking and reduce the proportion of animal fat in the diet.

Heart failure. Failure of the heart to pump blood around the body in adequate amounts. Heart failure may be caused by heart valve disease, high *blood pressure*, or damage to heart muscle following a *heart attack*. Symptoms include breathlessness, ankle swelling, cough and a bluish tinge to the lips.

TREATMENT. Careful medical treatment with heart stimulant and diuretic drugs is required in most cases, with bed rest and extra oxygen if this is needed to help breathing.

Leukaemia. Leukaemia is cancer of white blood cells. In most cases the causes are not known. It may develop suddenly or gradually. The symptoms include sore throat, fever, malaise, swollen glands and *anaemia*.

TREATMENT. The effectiveness of treatment depends on the type of leukaemia. Chemotherapy, using cancer-killing drugs, is the standard form of treatment.

Migraine. Severe recurring headaches often accompanied by nausea and disturbed vision. They are frequently one-sided. The causes are not known. The first signs of a migraine attack are often visual disorders such as a narrowed field of vision or flashing lights in front of the eyes. These effects are usually followed by a severe one-sided headache with a dislike of light and noise. In children recurrent attacks of vomiting may be the prelude to the development of typical migraine headaches as they grow older.

TREATMENT. Effervescent aspirin taken as soon as possible at the start of an attack is the most effective treatment. Lie down in a quiet place. Consult a doctor or an organization that specializes in the study of migraine for advice.

Paleness (pallor). Paleness indicates a reduced blood supply to the skin and may be a sign of cold, fatigue, recent illness, shock, or *anaemia*. If it persists, a doctor should be consulted.

Palpitations. The normal pulse rate in an adult at rest is about 70 or 80 beats a minute. Rapid regular beats (tachycardia) occur after exercise. An increased pulse rate can also be detected because of anxiety, smoking, an overactive thyroid, or some forms of heart disease. Slow, regular beats (bradycardia) are found in the trained athlete at rest. Bradycardia is also characteristic of an underactive thyroid. Missed beats (ventricular extrasystoles) may occasionally occur in the normal heart at rest. They are also caused by smoking and they may be a sign of heart disease. Irregular rapid beats (atrial fibrillation) and other irregularities are usually symptoms of heart disease. Any uncertainties about the condition of the heart should be discussed with a doctor as soon as possible. A thorough examination may be necessary to exclude the possibility of heart disease.

Blood and Heart Problems

Phlebitis. The inflammation of a vein, usually in the leg. It occurs most commonly as a result of childbirth, varicose veins, or an operation. The skin above the vein is tender and may be discoloured. Swelling of the leg may also occur. The inflammation may lead to the formation of a blood clot (thrombophlebitis).

TREATMENT. The leg should be firmly bandaged and the patient should be encouraged to move. Pain-killing and anti-inflammatory drugs may be prescribed. A hot compress placed on the inflamed area may help temporarily. Movement maintains the circulation in the affected limb.

Stroke. Sudden local or general paralysis due to injury of the brain or spinal cord. The common causes are an embolus blocking the blood supply to part of the brain, a haemorrhage in the brain, or thrombosis. A stroke may cause complete paralysis of one side of the body (hemiplegia) with loss of speech. A mild stroke, with momentary weakness, numbness, disorder of speech, and double vision may be followed by complete recovery. In all cases, a doctor should be informed.

Thrombosis. This occurs when a blood clot (thrombus) forms in part of the circulation and obstructs the blood flow. A haemorrhage may result if the clot causes the blood vessel to break. Thrombosis is likely to occur in blood vessel diseases such as *arteriosclerosis, phlebitis,* and *varicose veins*, or as a side-effect of smoking or use of the contraceptive pill. Any blood clotting is known as thrombosis and this is not necessarily pathological. Thrombosis of small veins always occurs around the site of an injury or infection.

A deep vein thrombosis usually occurs in the large veins deep in the muscles of the calf, thigh, or pelvis. It may occur after childbirth or an operation. The first signs may be ankle swelling or calf tenderness. A superficial venous thrombosis may occur in phlebitis. An arterial thrombosis is always serious. Coronary thrombosis leads to a *heart attack*. Thrombosis in an arteriosclerotic leg can lead to *gangrene*. In the brain a thrombosis causes a *stroke*.

TREATMENT. Thrombosis may be prevented by starting to take physical activity as soon as possible after an operation or, in certain cases, by the use of anticoagulant drugs. A deep vein thrombosis also requires treatment with anticoagulants but thrombophlebitis can be treated successfully with local heat and anti-rheumatic or pain-killing drugs if necessary.

Varicose veins. These are distorted, dilated veins usually found in the legs. They may be caused by damage to the valves following *thrombosis* or pregnancy or they may be due to a congenital defect in the valves. The pressure of blood, without the regulating effect of the valves, causes the veins to swell, to lose their elasticity and finally to remain dilated. Symptoms include aching legs, swelling and ulceration of the ankles, eczema, and sometimes thrombosis.

TREATMENT. Elastic stockings to support the veins and sitting with the legs raised may both help. An injection into the veins may be given to make them collapse completely. Six weeks' firm bandaging is required after this injection to make sure that the walls of the veins stick to each other. An operation to remove a vein or to cut it in various places to prevent back pressure in the damaged vein may be required. If a varicose vein bursts, see EMERGENCY FIRST AID, p.10.

Breast Problems

Breast Problems

Abscess. Breast abscesses usually occur during breast-feeding. They are caused by local infection, usually through the nipple, often because of a cracked nipple or lack of cleanliness. The symptoms are local pain, swelling and redness.

TREATMENT. Antibiotic treatment is required, with a doctor's prescription. In severe cases it may be necessary to undergo an operation to drain the abscess.

Babies' breasts. The breasts of new-born babies may sometimes produce milk. This occurs because milk-stimulating hormones from the mother's blood have passed into the baby's circulation and still remain to stimulate the baby's milk-secreting organs. This process will cease naturally within a few days.

Breast examination. A woman should examine her breasts regularly, preferably at the same time each month. Stand in front of a mirror, raise both arms sideways and look at the shape of the breasts to see if any unusual dimples occur. Then lie on the back and feel each breast gently with the flat of the hand. The outer half of each breast will have to be felt by the opposite hand. Pinching the breast with the thumb and fingers will feel only normal breast tissue, whereas the flat of the hand will detect abnormalities situated within the normal breast structure. If any abnormality is found or if you are in any doubt, consult a doctor at once.

Development. Breast development in adolescence is often associated with soreness. Most women have one breast slightly larger than the other and apparently uneven development is not abnormal. Approximately one adolescent boy in ten experiences tenderness in the breasts for a short period soon after puberty. Although this may cause anxiety, it is no more than a temporary effect and will disappear naturally.

Lump. A lump in the breast is not usually due to cancer but nevertheless it must be examined by a doctor. Various technical aids which include X-rays, mammography, and heat tests may help in making the correct diagnosis. It may be necessary to remove the lump for further examination with a microscope. Signs of cancer include puckering of the skin of the breast, red, weeping skin on the nipple and discharge from the nipple, some or all of which may be associated with a lump in the breast.

TREATMENT. If cancer is confirmed the breast can be removed (mastectomy) before further treatment with radiotherapy and with cancer-killing drugs (chemotherapy) is required.

Mastitis. An inflammation of the breast that may be caused by a breast *abscess* or by infection following *nipple disease*. The chief symptom is soreness of the breast tissue, more painful than the *tenderness* that is associated with menstruation and breast *development*. The breast will also appear red from the inflammation. Mastitis can occur during breast-feeding if the breast is infected through the nipple because of inadequate cleanliness.

TREATMENT. A doctor must be consulted. Antibiotic treatment may be necessary. Stop breast-feeding so that the infection is not passed on to the child.

Nipple disease. Sometimes a small amount of pale, milky fluid is produced during menstruation or when taking the contracep-

Chest and Respiratory Problems

tive pill. Soreness of the nipple may occur when breast feeding. Any other discharge or soreness must be reported to a doctor. If the skin of the nipple becomes red and appears moist without reason a doctor should also be consulted. Small sebaceous cysts may grow in the pigmented area of the nipple. These are not serious and can be removed.

Size. Breasts vary greatly in size and shape and the only definition of normal size or shape is that which is dictated by the fashion of the time. Nevertheless, breasts that are unusually large may cause discomfort as well as anxiety and breasts that are small may cause a feeling of a lack of femininity.

TREATMENT. In some cases, psychotherapy may help to alleviate anxiety. Cosmetic surgery to enlarge or to reduce breast size may also be considered, although it is expensive and is not guaranteed to be permanently effective.

Tenderness. Breast tenderness, swelling or tingling is common just before the time of the monthly period. If it is present for most of the month or if it is severe, consult a doctor. See also *Mastitis.*

Chest and Respiratory Problems

Altitude sickness (mountain sickness). The reaction of the body to a reduction of the oxygen content of the air at high altitudes. This occurs most commonly during rapid ascent to more than 8,000 feet (2,500 metres) although some people are not affected below 13,000 feet (4,000 metres). Symptoms include headache, *breathlessness,* palpitations, nausea, diarrhoea and extreme weakness.

TREATMENT. In mild cases, rest until the symptoms disappear. More severe cases require treatment with oxygen and diuretics and a return to lower altitudes. Patients with heart or lung disease should seek medical advice before ascending to high altitudes. Modern aeroplanes are pressurized to the equivalent of 5,000 feet (1,500 metres) so that there is no risk when they carry passengers at high altitudes.

Asthma. Asthma is a condition in which respiration is made difficult by spasms of the small breathing tubes (bronchioles). It is usually an inherited tendency that may be associated with eczema and hay fever, but it may also be due to infection, cold or anxiety. Complications include *bronchitis, pneumonia* and *emphysema.*

TREATMENT. Drugs may be used to cause the bronchioles to dilate. Some can be inhaled from special pressurized aerosols or sprays. Attacks may be prevented or stopped at an early stage by using bronchodilators or antihistamines or by the regular use of corticosteroid aerosols or sodium cromoglycate inhalers.

Blood, spitting of (haemoptysis). Any cold or minor respiratory infection may cause small blood vessels in the nose and throat to rupture, producing streaks of bright red blood in the *sputum.* This is normal and not serious. Dental problems, such as infected gums (gingivitis) or teeth may also cause minor bleeding.

Bright red blood coughed up from the lungs may be a serious symptom but it is most commonly associated with *bronchitis.* If it occurs alone it may indicate lung scarring (bronchiectasis), tuberculosis, cancer of the lung or a blood clot (embolus) from elsewhere that has lodged in the lung.

77

Chest and Respiratory Problems

TREATMENT. If the bleeding is serious a doctor must be consulted immediately so that the cause can be diagnosed.

Breathlessness. If this is acute and occurs for the first time it may be that something has been inhaled. Sudden breathlessness may be due to rupture of a lung, a blood clot (embolus), acute heart failure from a heart attack or an infection such as *croup* or *pneumonia*. Recurrent attacks of acute breathlessness are symptoms of *asthma*, heart failure or acute anxiety. Recent and gradual breathlessness may be due to a variety of causes such as anaemia, anxiety, asthma, cancer of a lung or chronic heart failure. Persistent breathlessness occurs in *bronchitis* with *emphysema* and in lung diseases such as pneumonconiosis, which is often caused by industrial conditions such as those encountered in coal mining and quarrying.

Bronchitis, acute. Acute bronchitis is indicated by the onset of a cough, often with thick sputum, and is associated with pain behind the breast bone, fever and malaise. It often develops after a *cold*.

TREATMENT. Stop smoking and consult a doctor. Hot steam inhalations with menthol, a sedative cough mixture at night, an expectorant during the day, a warm room, a light diet and sufficient to drink will all help recovery. Antibiotics will be given if the doctor considers them necessary. The illness usually lasts less than a week if the patient is careful but a cough may continue for a further two weeks.

Bronchitis, chronic. *Asthma, smoking,* industrial pollution or repeated attacks of acute bronchitis will damage the lining of the breathing tubes (bronchi) and will prevent the normal drainage of mucus from the lungs. Because this drainage is slower at night a morning cough, to clear the sputum, will generally occur. Coughing may also take place throughout the day. Recurring attacks of acute with chronic bronchitis need immediate antibiotic treatment.

TREATMENT. Stop smoking and avoid a polluted environment. Breathing exercises help to keep lungs clear of mucus.

Catarrh. Inflammation of the membranes of the nose with a thick mucus discharge. It may be caused by recurrent colds, vasomotor rhinitis, chronic sinusitis, nasal polyps, allergy, dust irritation, *smoking,* or a deviated nasal septum. In children it may be aggravated by enlarged adenoids.

Chest, tightness in the. This describes a feeling similar to that occurring after strenuous exercise. It may be a symptom of respiratory illnesses, such as *asthma* or *pneumonia,* or it may be caused by anxiety or indigestion.

Cold, common. Symptoms of a cold may be caused by any one of at least 40 different viruses. Colds are most infectious while they are developing. Symptoms include sneezing, sore throat, red eyes, general malaise and slight muscle aching, followed by a running nose for two or three days and then *catarrh* for a further week.

TREATMENT. Antihistamines, aspirin, throat lozenges and nasal sprays may help to control the symptoms. Stay in a warm atmosphere for the acute stage, preferably away from others to stop the spread of infection.

Cough. A noisy clearing of irritation from the respiratory passages. The irritation may be caused by *catarrh* from the nose flowing into the throat (post-nasal drip), by throat infections,

Chest and Respiratory Problems

by *asthma,* by lung infections such as *bronchitis* and *pneumonia,* by irritation of the diaphragm from stomach disorders such as *gastritis* or by a nervous habit or anxiety. See also *Infectious Illnesses: Whooping cough.*

Croup. Croup is a harsh, barking cough combined with a rough, grating sound (stridor) that accompanies breathing. It is most common in small children in whom the respiratory tubes are narrow. Partial obstruction of a child's vocal cords can occur as a result of infection or inhalation of a foreign body. Croup also occurs in minor respiratory illnesses but is serious only if the child has difficulty breathing.

TREATMENT. A warm, humid atmosphere relieves the symptoms. Children also need reassurance. Antihistamines may help and breathing is easier if the child is propped up on pillows. It is often more alarming to parents than to the child, who is likely to fall asleep despite the rough breathing.

Emphysema. A serious reduction in the internal surface area of the lungs. This occurs because the small sponge-like structures (alveoli) that fill the lungs and provide the large internal surface area are damaged and collapse. This damage is usually caused by the coughing of chronic *bronchitis* and *asthma.* Emphysema causes *breathlessness* on exercise.

Laryngitis. Acute laryngitis is caused by a throat infection that affects the vocal cords. Chronic laryngitis occurs if the vocal cords continue to be used during an acute attack. The inflammation is aggravated by smoke and alcohol.

TREATMENT. Rinse the mouth regularly and gargle with an antiseptic mouth wash. Try to speak as softly and as little as possible. If the symptoms persist, consult a doctor.

Pleurisy. An infection of the pleural membrane that lines the chest cavity and surrounds the lungs. Inflammation causes extreme pain in the chest when breathing, coughing or moving. Pleurisy may be caused by *pneumonia,* cancer, a blood clot or an infection from a wound.

TREATMENT. Consult a doctor immediately so that the correct treatment can be given. Sit propped up in bed with a hot pad over the painful side. Antibiotics will probably be required and a sedative cough mixture and pain-killing drugs may also be prescribed.

Pneumonia. A serious infection of lung tissue. It occurs most commonly as bronchopneumonia which may develop as an extension of *bronchitis.* Lobar pneumonia, an infection of an anatomical segment of the lungs, may also occur. Pneumonia is caused by a variety of bacteria or viruses. The symptoms include *cough,* fever and *pleurisy.* These may develop suddenly or gradually following a *cold* or bronchitis.

TREATMENT. Appropriate antibiotics are necessary, and breathing exercises, steam inhalations, pain-killing drugs, and cough mixtures also help. It is essential to stop smoking. Pneumonia is particularly serious in the elderly and in those suffering from any other serious illness.

Smoking. The effects of smoking on health are numerous. Those who smoke 25 cigarettes a day have a death rate from chronic *bronchitis* that is 20 times greater than non-smokers. Cancer of the lung kills one man in seven in the 55-60 age group. Smoking increases the dangers of heart attack and arteriosclerosis, doubles the risk of cancer of the bladder and is also a significant factor in some forms of blindness, ging-

Chest and Respiratory Problems

ivitis, and peptic ulcers. In women, smoking increases the probability of stillbirth and miscarriage and the birth weight of babies born to women who smoke is lower than average.

TREATMENT. Discuss the habit with a doctor. To stop smoking requires determination. The doctor may recommend some drugs that can help. The physical withdrawal takes about two weeks, during which time the symptoms described above may become severe. After two weeks any further symptoms are probably psychological in origin.

Tracheitis. An inflammation of the trachea, associated with *laryngitis* and *bronchitis.* Symptoms include coughing that causes pain behind the upper part of the breastbone and sometimes a mild fever.

TREATMENT. Steam inhalations, cough mixtures and a warm, humid room may relieve the symptoms until recovery. If the inflammation persists or becomes too uncomfortable, a doctor should be consulted.

Children's Problems

Bedwetting (nocturnal enuresis). Bedwetting is common in children below the age of three. Most children are completely dry by the age of six but there are some who are still occasional bedwetters in their early teens. If bedwetting starts again some time after it originally ceased, there may be an emotional cause, such as anxiety.

TREATMENT. Wait for natural improvement. Offering careful encouragement, with charts showing which have been the dry nights, may also help.

Blue baby. A newborn baby may have a slightly blue appearance. This is caused by poorly oxygenated blood in the circulation and is usually the result of difficulties in breathing immediately after birth. The blueness is apparent in the lips, the earlobes and the tips of the fingers. In certain cases the blueness does not disappear, and the tongue may also appear blue. This suggests a more serious defect in the respiratory system or in the heart. The hole-in-the-heart baby is a blue baby of this kind. Such defects must be repaired by surgery either at once or when the child is about one year old.

Bow-legs (genu varum). When babies start walking, between 12 and 18 months of age, there is an outward curvature of the legs. The legs gradually become straighter and even *knock-kneed* (genu valgum) at the age of about three years before they become naturally straight in the fourth year of life.

TREATMENT. There is not normally any need to treat this process as it will correct itself naturally. Rarely, bow-legs in a growing child are due to rickets. In such cases vitamin D supplements will strengthen the growing bone.

Breath-holding attack. Such attacks usually occur between the ages of one and four. They are usually started by a sudden shock, accident or fit of temper. The child cries out and holds its breath for about 20 seconds, then turns blue in the face and falls down, apparently unconscious. Recovery time is about 15 seconds. These attacks resemble epilepsy but anger or fright at the onset indicate the difference.

TREATMENT. Ignore the attack if possible and do not give way to the child's temper. Patience and understanding are necessary until this condition improves naturally. Discuss the problem with a doctor.

Children's Problems

Colic. In babies this is a sign of abdominal pain. The baby cries, draws up its knees and is clearly distressed. Colic is often due to *wind* and failure to get rid of it after a feed. Three-month colic commonly occurs in the evenings at this age and is probably due to a variety of causes such as a rushed evening feed, wind, boredom, or the change in diet as solids are introduced. It settles in time and may be helped by cuddling the baby or by giving an antispasm medicine obtained from a doctor. Colic may also indicate serious problems such as a hernia, a twisted bowel or intussusception, in which case the baby continues to cry and the pains obviously become more severe. A doctor must be consulted. In an older child colicky pain may result from the wrong food, an intestinal illness or possibly appendicitis.

Constipation. Difficulty in defecation due to hard faeces. This is common in children because of slight dehydration. Sometimes it may be caused by feeds made in too strong a solution. Occasionally constipation is caused by a tear of the skin of the anus, which causes pain and bleeding when passing faeces. TREATMENT. Give extra fluid and, if the child is old enough, fruit and vegetables. A glycerin suppository for infants or, in older children, milk of magnesia may be needed.

Crying. All babies cry. At first it is their only way of expressing themselves. They may cry for food, attention, because of discomfort, or because of pain from *colic*. Older babies may cry out of boredom. Let them watch you at work around the home and let them feel part of the family in the evening. Younger children cry because of frustration or temper, pain or fear.

Diarrhoea. In babies this describes stools that are more fluid than usual. The yellow porridge-like stool of the breast-fed baby may occur once a day and that of the bottle-fed baby several times a day. Green stools are an indication that the intestinal contents have passed through more quickly than usual and the green bile has not had time to change colour. Diarrhoea alone is not serious provided that the baby appears well and is eating and drinking normally. It may also be caused by an inappropriate diet. Dehydration may occur if the baby is not drinking enough or starts *vomiting* and this can be dangerous, especially in the very young. Diarrhoea with *colic,* particularly if there is blood in the stool, requires urgent medical attention.

Fits and convulsions. Fits may involve a sudden loss of consciousness, twitching, and shaking with teeth clenched, sometimes frothing at the mouth, and rolling eyes. Breathing is usually noisy and rapid. Involuntary urination may occur. A fit (seizure) commonly lasts for about 20 to 30 seconds before the child recovers consciousness. After a fit a child usually falls into a normal sleep. In children fits are commonly caused by high fever, but they may also be due to a brain infection such as meningitis or encephalitis, or to epilepsy. A doctor must be consulted at once. TREATMENT. During a fit, hold the child to prevent smothering or injury. If there is fever, cool the skin and give aspirin and a cold drink on recovery. Take the child's temperature every hour and sponge the skin if the temperature rises above 103°F (39°C). Further treatment will be given by the doctor and investigations in hospital may be necessary when the child has recovered.

81

Children's Problems

Knock-knee (genu valgum). This is a common deformity, at the age of about three or four years, following *bow-legs*. There is no need to treat it as it will almost always improve naturally. If it is still present when the child is ten years old, surgical treatment may be required.

Masturbation. Most babies sooner or later find pleasure in touching their own genitals. Boys will have erections due to a full bladder as well as from masturbation. Rocking movements that rub the genitals often produce a flushed, almost trance-like state followed by relaxation and sleep. This does no harm. The baby or child should not be reprimanded or punished but, if possible, should be distracted by some more sociable occupation. Most children grow out of this stage when young and return to it at puberty. In rare cases, compulsive masturbation, to the exclusion of normal life, is a sign of insecurity and anxiety. This will require skilled psychiatric help for the child and the family.

Nappy rash (diaper rash). The chapping and chafing of a baby's buttocks and groins due to the dampness of wet nappies combined with the irritating effects of urine on the skin. It may also be associated with atopic eczema or with irritation of the skin by soap or detergent in the nappies. Occasionally moniliasis or an infection such as impetigo may occur.

TREATMENT. Always rinse nappies well and change them frequently. Leave the baby without nappies whenever possible. Zinc oxide and castor oil cream or a proprietary cream will clear mild rashes. Severe rashes should be seen by a doctor as antifungal treatment may be required.

Night terrors. Babies may wake terrified and screaming during the night. If old enough, a child may be able to describe a nightmare but often it is unable to do so. Night terrors may occur frequently for a period of time and then cease. At some time or another they are common in most young children. They may be due to an active imagination or to more deep-seated anxiety and insecurity.

TREATMENT. Reassurance and cuddling from a parent until the child is sleepy again is the only immediate treatment. It is rarely necessary to consult a doctor unless night terrors recur very frequently.

Puberty. Puberty is the stage of growth during which the secondary sexual characteristics develop. A girl's breasts develop and her body acquires the shape of a young woman. A boy's voice deepens and hair starts to grow on his face, arms, legs, and chest and in the pubic region. Menstruation and sperm formation start at about the same stage of development so that from this time reproduction is possible. Puberty is associated with the psychological changes of adolescence. These affect not only sexuality but also the adolescent's relationships with parents and other adults.

Sleep-walking. Sleep-walking occurs most commonly between the ages of five and ten. It is not dangerous and the sleep-walker seems to retain normal cautiousness. Its causes are not clearly known, but underlying emotional insecurity or anxiety may be the causes in some children.

TREATMENT. Sleep-walking usually ceases naturally so there is no need for treatment. Take the child back to bed. There is no harm in waking a sleep-walker. Do not be anxious yourself as this will only worry the child.

Spina bifida. This is a congenital deformity of the lower part of the spine due to failure of the vertebrae to join. It may be so slight that it is noticed only on an X-ray, or so severe that none of the tissues over the lower part of the back have joined and the covering of the spinal cord is exposed. The severe form is often associated with hydrocephalus, a condition in which the brain of the child swells because the normal circulation of its fluid is blocked. As the brain swells, the skull also increases in size. The causes of these congenital abnormalities are not known. Spina bifida can often be detected by special tests in early pregnancy. In the mild form there may be no symptoms. Paralysis of the legs and bladder may occur in the severe form and meningitis may develop because the membranes surrounding the spinal cord are exposed.

Teething. Some babies are born with teeth and others do not produce them until they are more than one year old. Teething usually causes little trouble apart from occasional slight irritation and apparent discomfort. A teething ring may help this. Children usually have all their milk teeth by the age of 30 months and start losing them, when the permanent teeth arrive, from the age of about six years.

Thumb sucking. Thumb sucking is normal in most new-born babies, and soon stops. It is likely to return at the age of about six months and is a habit that seems to comfort and reassure a child and often helps with sleep. It usually ceases by the age of four or five.

Vomiting. Many babies regurgitate after a feed. This is not harmful and may be a sign of contentment. Occasionally an older baby vomits regularly after a meal but gains weight and is clearly well. This too is a habit, often in a lively, cheerful baby. Vomiting may occur during a cold if mucus is swallowed and then vomited, or following a severe coughing bout, particularly with whooping cough. It may also occur as a part of a generalized illness associated with fever, such as a middle ear infection (otitis media), or with *diarrhoea*. If it is caused by intestinal obstruction, *colic* and abdominal swelling will also be apparent. Rarely, vomiting may indicate an allergy to cow's milk.

TREATMENT. Decide whether the vomiting is due to regurgitation or whether it is associated with a cold or more serious problem. Dehydration, usually due to vomiting associated with diarrhoea, is a potential danger. Generalized infections and intestinal obstructions need rapid medical attention. Less serious vomiting is treated by resting the stomach. Stop meals and give small amounts of water every hour and increase this quantity only when the vomiting has stopped. As soon as the baby has started to drink properly, half-strength milk and then solids can be given.

Wind. Air swallowing occurs naturally in babies during feeding. It is increased by too small a hole in the teat. A baby likes to be cuddled and played with after a feed and this is the time when excess wind may be burped up. See also three-month *Colic*.

Ear Problems

Bat ear. A slight congenital deformity that makes the outer ear stand out noticeably from the head.

TREATMENT. Cosmetic surgery, between the ages of four and six, may be performed if the appearance is worrying.

Ear Problems

Deafness. A difficulty with hearing that may be caused by blockage or damage to the outer or middle ear, or by damage to the nerve or the cochlea. A sudden onset of deafness is always alarming and until a doctor is consulted nose drops and steam inhalations may relieve middle ear blockage. Do not use ear drops. Sudden deafness and pain, with or without discharge, is usually caused by an infection of the outer tube to the eardrum (*otitis externa*), an infection of the middle ear (*otitis media*) or to sudden changes in atmospheric pressure. Sudden deafness without pain may be caused by *wax*, blockage of the middle ear by catarrh, a nerve infection following mumps, by a small haemorrhage into the cochlea, or by damage from extremely loud noise. A gradual onset of deafness is usually caused by wax, by repeated exposure to gunfire or noisy machinery, by ageing, or by a family tendency to deafness such as otosclerosis (which affects the three small vibrating bones of the middle ear). Deafness at birth may be hereditary or the result of a maternal infection, such as German measles, during the first three months of pregnancy.
TREATMENT. In all cases, the earlier a diagnosis is made the better the chance of curing deafness and, in the young, of educating the child correctly and teaching it to speak in order to avoid dumbness.

Earache. Pain in or just behind the ear. This is normally due to a boil or infection of the outer tube (*otitis externa*), an infection of the middle ear (*otitis media*), to *mastoiditis*, to pain from the jaw joint, or to pain that originates in and is referred from the teeth or throat.
TREATMENT. Use pain-killing drugs such as aspirin. Do not use ear drops until you have received a doctor's advice on the cause of the pain.

Ear discharging. A discharge from the ear may indicate an infection of the outer tube of the ear or it may come from an infected middle ear, if the eardrum has ruptured.
TREATMENT. Do not get the ear wet and do not use ear drops until you have received a doctor's advice.

Mastoiditis. An acute or chronic infection of the bone behind the ear, usually caused by the spread of infection from *otitis media*.
TREATMENT. Consult a doctor. Large doses of antibiotics usually cure mastoiditis but occasionally an operation (mastoidectomy) is needed to remove the infected bone.

Ménière's disease. A disease caused by an intermittent increase of fluid pressure in the inner ear. It usually occurs in people over the age of about 40. In one case out of four both ears become involved. The cause is not known. Symptoms include intermittent attacks of giddiness, buzzing in the ear, nausea, vomiting, and gradually increasing *deafness* over a number of years. Each attack lasts from minutes to hours but the buzzing can continue all the time and lead to depression.
TREATMENT. It may help to lie down and take antinausea medication. In the long-term treatment, a variety of drugs are used and sometimes an operation can cure the disease.

Otitis externa. An infection of the outer tube of the ear. It may be caused by a form of eczema, by swimming, particularly in hot climates, by scratching the ears with the finger nails, and occasionally by excess *wax*. Symptoms include itching, a slight discharge from the ear, *earache*, *deafness*, or fever,

84

Eye Problems

TREATMENT. Do not scratch the ear and keep water out. Consult a doctor for the appropriate treatment with antibiotic ear drops. Clean excess wax from the ears.

Otitis media. An infection of the middle ear. It is usually associated with a cold and catarrh blocking the Eustachian tube, with acute tonsillitis, or with flying or diving while suffering from catarrh. Symptoms include *earache, deafness,* fever, and a discharge if the eardrum bursts.

TREATMENT. Immediate treatment is necessary, using nose drops, antihistamines and pain-killing drugs followed by antibiotics from a doctor. Do not use ear drops. Inadequate treatment may lead to *mastoiditis* or deafness.

Wax. Ear wax is a sticky, orange-brown secretion from the external tube of the ear which may block it and cause irritation or *deafness.*

TREATMENT. Consult a doctor. Do not attempt to extract a plug of wax yourself as you risk pushing it farther in and possibly damaging the eardrum.

Eye Problems

Astigmatism. Distortion of the shape of objects caused by a fault in the cornea or the lens of the eye. It can be corrected by wearing appropriate spectacles.

Blindness. The loss of clear vision in one or both eyes. There may still be an ability to recognize light and dark and moving shadows. Sudden blindness in both eyes is very rare and usually follows an accident or a stroke. Sudden blindness in one eye indicates blockage of the artery to the eye from an embolus or a thrombosis, or detachment of the retina, or possibly an inflammation of the nerve, as in multiple sclerosis or polyneuritis. Momentary blindness may occur during the onset of migraine, or it may be caused by a small embolus passing through the artery to the eye. Low blood pressure at the moment of fainting may also cause momentary blindness (black-out). Gradual blindness may indicate *glaucoma,* a *cataract,* the degeneration of the retina, high blood pressure, diabetes, or recurrent ulcers of the outer surface of the eye.

TREATMENT. This depends on the cause and requires a thorough examination by a doctor to exclude general problems as well as specific eye diseases.

Cataract. An opacity that forms in the lens. At first it produces mistiness of vision but, ultimately, *blindness* may occur. A person may be born with a cataract, sometimes caused by the mother having German measles during the first 12 weeks of pregnancy. It commonly occurs in the elderly due to natural degeneration of the lens, and can be treated by removing the damaged lens and using special spectacles or contact lenses.

Conjunctivitis. An infection or inflammation of the clear tissue that covers the outer surface of the eye (the conjunctiva). Conjunctivitis causes watering from the eye, redness, and sometimes the discharge of pus with irritation and occasionally slight pain. Acute conjunctivitis often occurs with a cold or minor virus respiratory illness. More severe attacks are known as pink eye, caused by infectious bacteria that may develop into an epidemic in certain circumstances. Conjunctivitis also occurs with measles and scarlet fever. Chronic conjunctivitis is caused by irritation from dusty or polluted atmospheres and is often associated with allergies.

Eye Problems

TREATMENT. Do not rub an infected eye as this is likely to transmit infection to the other eye. Do not wear a patch over the eye as this may increase the severity of the infection. Consult a doctor for the appropriate treatment.

Glaucoma. This is a condition in which the pressure of the fluid in the eye increases. This pressure prevents the normal circulation of blood, damages the nerve cells that respond to light and ultimately causes *blindness*. Symptoms are a gradual or intermittent deterioration of vision, rings or haloes around bright lights, a red eye and severe eye pain, sometimes accompanied by vomiting.

TREATMENT. Careful medical supervision is required to detect pressure changes in the eye. The acute, painful, red eye with blurred vision must be reported immediately to a doctor.

Gritty feeling in the eye. This is only rarely due to dust or a foreign body. Usually it is a symptom of *conjunctivitis*.

Iritis. Inflammation or infection of the coloured area of the eye. There are many different causes. Iritis is usually accompanied by some pain, by blurring of vision and by intolerance of light.

TREATMENT. Iritis requires urgent medical attention.

Itching. Itching of the eyes may be due to mild *conjunctivitis*, to an inflammation of the eyelids (blepharitis), or an allergy.

Lids, sore and swollen. This is commonly associated with *conjunctivitis, styes* and, sometimes, with cysts on the eyelid. It may also indicate excessive tiredness, or be a reaction to a smoky atmosphere.

Lids, twitching. This commonly occurs on the outer side of the eyelid as an uncontrollable flickering (tic) of the muscles of the face. It is a symptom of anxiety or fatigue. It is not usually serious and should improve spontaneously. If it does not, a doctor should be consulted.

Long-sightedness (hypermetropia). This is indicated if there is excellent distance vision but difficulty with seeing close objects. It may cause headaches, and watering and aching eyes when reading. It occurs as an inherited tendency, and can be corrected by spectacles.

Short-sightedness (myopia). Difficulty in seeing distant objects indicates myopia. Short-sightedness is considered to be an inherited tendency. It is corrected by wearing spectacles.

Stye. A stye is an infected hair follicle in the eyelid. It often occurs in children, and may be associated with *conjunctivitis*.

TREATMENT. Bathe the eye with warm water several times a day. This will encourage the stye to discharge. Do not squeeze or rub an infected eye.

Foot and Hand Problems

Athlete's foot. Athlete's foot is a chronic, fungal infection of the superficial skin of the foot, especially between the toes and on the soles. Symptoms include scaling, soreness, itching, and cracked and softened skin. The cracks may lead to inflammation of the underlying tissue. The condition is easily transmitted in public swimming baths, school gyms and other places where people walk bare-foot. Careful drying between the toes is an effective method of preventing this fungal infection spreading.

TREATMENT. Anti-fungal preparations from a chemist may clear athlete's foot but if these do not work, consult a doctor.

Foot and Hand Problems

Blister. Blisters are caused by part of a shoe rubbing the skin of the foot and occur particularly as a result of long-distance marching or hiking. Not only the fluid-filled blister itself but also the surrounding skin is likely to be painful.

TREATMENT. Do not burst a blister, but keep it covered with a clean, protective pad. Harden the affected skin with surgical spirit and rest the foot if possible.

Bunion. A bunion is a swelling over the side of the big toe joint, usually associated with a deformity which makes the toe point towards the other toes. Bunions are caused by tight-fitting, pointed shoes, particularly those with high heels that throw the weight forwards. As the shoe rubs, the toe is twisted out of position and the skin thickens. A small fluid-containing area (bursa) forms in the tissue around the joint which swells to produce the bunion.

TREATMENT. In mild cases, it is sufficient to wear wide-toed, low-heeled shoes. If pain continues, a chiropodist should be consulted. The use of felt pads to separate the big toe from the others will prevent further pressure. In severe cases, in which there is considerable deformity and arthritis of the toe, an operation is needed.

Chilblain. Cold and damp conditions are liable to cause the hands, fingers, feet and toes and sometimes the ears to become inflamed. The inflammation produces red swellings that may be itchy and painful when the affected part becomes warm. Chilblains resemble a mild form of frostbite and if untreated the damaged tissue may ulcerate.

TREATMENT. Do not rub the chilblain but warm the area gradually. Pain-killing drugs may be used in treatment. In all but the mildest cases a doctor should be consulted.

Corn. A concentric thickening of the skin on the toe or foot caused by a tight shoe. It is often tender.

TREATMENT. Protect the corn from further pressure with a circular corn pad. Corn-removing solutions soften the skin and so may allow the hard centre of the corn to drop out or be removed.

Flat foot. A condition in which the whole surface of the sole of the foot is in contact with the ground, and in which the normal arch beneath the foot is lacking. The condition may be due to long periods of standing, to a congenital defect, to muscle weakness, or to paralysis following poliomyelitis. Children normally have flat feet for the first few years of life.

TREATMENT. If the foot does not develop normally exercises or a support for the sole may help.

Heberden's nodes. Cartilagenous and bony nodules that occur near the end joints of mildly osteo-arthritic fingers, particularly in the elderly. Sometimes the nodules may be tender and inflamed but usually the inflammation settles without treatment in two or three weeks.

Toe-nail, ingrowing. This usually affects the big toes and is often caused by pressure from tight shoes and incorrect nail-cutting. The ingrowing nail cuts into the side of the toe forming a fissure which may become infected, especially where there is a lack of cleanliness.

TREATMENT. Infection should be treated by applying strips of gauze soaked in antiseptic liquid to the side of the nail, but if it continues, consult a doctor. Prevent recurrences by cutting the nails so that the corners do not stick into the skin.

Foot and Hand Problems

Whitlow. An infection around the nails at the ends of the fingers or toes. The symptoms include pain and swelling followed by the formation of pus. It is commonly caused by nail-biting or by working with the hands in hot water or in unhygienic conditions. It may also be due to moniliasis (candidiasis), an infection caused by a species of the fungus Candida.

TREATMENT. If the infection is severe, a minor operation under local anaesthetic is required to open and clean the wound. Antifungal creams will prevent moniliasis.

Gynaecological Problems

Abortion. A term commonly used to refer to the deliberate termination of a *pregnancy*. The term is used medically to describe a spontaneous abortion that occurs before the 28th week of pregnancy. Deliberate abortions are sometimes performed as a form of birth control. In most cases this method is used only if it is considered that continuation of the pregnancy would endanger the life or health of the mother. An abortion can be performed using a special suction apparatus if a menstrual period is a few days overdue and during the first three months of pregnancy, or by a simple operation of dilatation and curettage (*D and C*). After this stage prostaglandins may be used to induce uterine contractions resembling those of labour. Certain cases may require an abdominal operation. See also *Miscarriage*.

Bleeding. Bleeding from the vagina is normal if it is due to *periods*. Abnormal, unexpected bleeding may be associated with *menstrual disorders,* the *menopause* or contraception, particularly if the contraceptive pill or an intrauterine device is used. If a woman is pregnant bleeding probably indicates a threatened *miscarriage*. In all cases, unusual bleeding should be reported to a doctor, particularly if it occurs after the menopause, and this should be done as soon as possible if the bleeding is severe.

Contraceptive problems. Reliable contraceptive methods for women include the diaphragm (Dutch cap), intrauterine devices (IUDs), contraceptive pills and sterilization. There are no problems associated with the diaphragm if it is properly used. Nevertheless it is inconvenient to use and this may account for the occasions when this method fails. IUDs can cause pain and heavy menstruation, particularly in women who have not had children, and, in rare cases, infection. The contraceptive pill is particularly suitable for young women. Side-effects of the pill in younger women are commonly limited to slight vaginal discharge, nausea, and possibly some weight gain. Problems arising from the pill become more serious with increasing age and alternative methods may be preferred for women over the age of 35. Sterilization may lead to some psychological problems due to regret for having had it done, owing to the fact that it is usually irreversible. For additional information on contraceptives, see *Urogenital Problems: Contraception*.

D and C (dilatation and curettage). A simple operation, performed under general anaesthetic, in which the neck (cervix) of the uterus is stretched open (dilated) sufficiently to admit a small instrument, a curette, into the uterus to scrape out the contents. D and C is usually performed to investigate *menstrual disorders*.

Gynaecological Problems

False pains. Throughout pregnancy the uterus is gently contracting and relaxing. Towards the end of the pregnancy these irregular contractions become stronger and may cause backache and lower abdominal pains, resembling those of *labour*, particularly at night.

TREATMENT. Mild pain-killing and sedative drugs may be required. Above all the woman needs reassurance that these pains are really "false".

Fibroid. A tumour of fibrous connective tissue that develops in the muscular wall of the uterus. More than one fibroid is usually found. Fibroids occur more commonly in childless women and only rarely indicate cancer. Symptoms include heavy *periods* and sometimes pressure on the bladder that causes frequent urination. Fibroids rarely cause pain unless they become infected.

TREATMENT. Nothing need be done unless the symptoms are troublesome or the fibroids are large. Individual fibroids can be removed (fibromectomy or myomectomy) but others may grow later. Fibroids may disturb the lining of the uterus and prevent conception, so their removal is necessary if a woman wishes to become pregnant.

Flooding. Profuse menstrual bleeding, usually so severe that it is difficult to absorb with external sanitary towels. It may be of brief duration or prolonged. It can recur with each period or it can occur unexpectedly between periods. Flooding is usually caused by hormonal disturbance, particularly a few years before the *menopause*, or by anxiety. It may also be associated with *fibroids, salpingitis,* or *miscarriage.*

Labour. The process by which a baby is born. Labour lasts 8 to 20 hours for the first baby and usually less for subsequent births. Labour has three stages. The first is the longest stage, lasting from the onset of labour to the moment when the neck (cervix) of the uterus is fully open. In the second stage the baby moves from the uterus through the pelvis. The second stage includes the birth. The third stage lasts until the afterbirth is expelled. The onset of labour is usually accompanied by backache, regular uterine contractions that become painful, and the appearance of blood and mucus. At this stage the mother should go to hospital or call a doctor or midwife for skilled medical care at home. The rupture of the amniotic membranes, with loss of the "waters", may occur at the onset or later in the course of labour.

Lightening. This usually occurs in the last few weeks of *pregnancy* when the baby's head settles deep into the mother's pelvis. Lightening leaves more room in the mother's abdomen and this gives a feeling of comfort. It may be accompanied by the need to urinate frequently because of pressure on the bladder.

Menopause. This usually occurs between the ages of 45 and 55 and signifies the end of menstruation. The menopause is also known as the female climacteric. It may be preceded by several months of irregular menstruation and it is associated with other symptoms caused by the gradual hormonal changes that occur at this age. Depression, loss of sexual interest, flushes, palpitations or tension may also occur.

TREATMENT. Many women do not have any symptoms that worry or concern them and do not need treatment. Others may find the symptoms distressing and a doctor can he   with

Gynaecological Problems

various treatments, including hormone replacement therapy. Any vaginal bleeding that occurs more than six months after the last period may indicate a serious disorder, such as cancer, and a doctor must be consulted.

Menstrual disorders. Irregular bleeding, bleeding that occurs too frequently or too heavily (*flooding*), or the absence of periods (amenorrhoea) is usually due to hormonal disorders. Amenorrhoea may be due to pregnancy, early *menopause*, anorexia nervosa, anxiety, or any severe or prolonged illness. It may also occur after oral contraception has been stopped. TREATMENT. Discuss the symptoms with a doctor. If menstruation has stopped, have a *pregnancy test* to exclude early pregnancy. If necessary, hormonal treatment or a *D and C* operation may be required. Amenorrhoea is only rarely a symptom of a more serious complaint and usually it is best to wait until menstruation restarts naturally.

Miscarriage. A lay term for *abortion*, the loss of a baby before the 28th week of pregnancy, usually in the first three months. At least 10% of all pregnancies end in a miscarriage. Most are due to an abnormality in the fetus, but some are due to hormonal imbalance and a few to weakness in the neck of the womb, illness or severe trauma. The principal symptom is vaginal bleeding during pregnancy. This is abnormal and must be regarded as a sign of a threatened miscarriage. If there is pain and loss of tissue, miscarriage is inevitable. TREATMENT. If there is heavy bleeding, possibly accompanied by backache and cramp-like pain, lie down on a plastic sheet covered with towelling and have an extra towel available to staunch further bleeding. Inform a doctor at once. If heavy bleeding continues the doctor will arrange urgent admission to hospital. The doctor should also be consulted if there is light bleeding without pain. Remain in bed until no further bleeding has occurred for at least 24 hours. Initial bleeding is bright red but this will become brown, indicating old blood, as it settles.

Morning sickness. This affects about 50% of women during early pregnancy. It is seldom severe but may be aggravated by anxiety or travelling.
TREATMENT. Small meals eaten at frequent intervals, and a drink of milk and a biscuit before moving in the morning, prevent an excess of gastric secretions. Certain drugs taken in early pregnancy may harm a fetus and a doctor must be consulted before anti-nausea drugs are used.

Periods (menstruation). The onset (menarche) of periods is usually between the ages of 10 and 14. They cease at the *menopause*, between the ages of 45 and 55. At first they may be irregular, and vary in length and amount of bleeding. After two or three years most girls settle into a regular rhythm. The first day of bleeding is the first day of the menstrual cycle, the period of bleeding lasts four to six days and the next cycle begins with the onset of the next period. Cycles generally last between 26 and 30 days. Some girls may have a longer (eg six-week) or a shorter (eg three-week) cycle.

Ovulation, the production of the egg, usually occurs in the middle of the cycle, 14 days before menstruation begins. Periods may occur without ovulation and it is also possible to ovulate without having had a period for some time.

When the periods first start, external sanitary towels are

Gynaecological Problems

usually found to be easiest to use. A girl should be instructed in their use and her mother should advise her before the event as the first period can be frightening if it occurs unexpectedly. When periods are regular, and the girl is physically larger, internal tampons are frequently used. The use of internal tampons requires a little practice and care. After a period, douching with warm water or a warm weak solution of bicarbonate of soda is unlikely to do harm but stronger chemicals should not be used. Reasonable external washing and careful drying are all that are required.

Periods, painful (dysmenorrhoea). In older women pain may be due to *salpingitis,* to an inflammation of the uterus or it may be associated with *premenstrual tension.* Characteristically, the pain lasts throughout the period. Between the ages of 15 and 25 cramping pain in the lower abdomen, sometimes with backache and pain down either side of the thighs, may start 24 hours before, and last for 24 to 48 hours after, the start of the period.

TREATMENT. A doctor should be consulted. Treatment should be started before the pain begins, if possible, and should continue throughout the period. Do not wait for the pain to return or become severe. Many women are helped by simple pain-killing drugs taken every four hours. The contraceptive pill may have a beneficial side-effect in stopping painful periods. In some cases, a *D and C* operation may be required.

Pregnancy. Pregnancy lasts for about 280 days from the moment of conception (fertilization of the ovum by the sperm) in the Fallopian tube until the end of the second stage of *labour* when the baby is born. The expected day of delivery (EDD) is calculated as nine months and seven days after the first day of the last period. During the first three months indications of pregnancy include swollen and tender breasts, *morning sickness,* and minimal weight gain. In the second three months, *quickening* occurs with gradual weight gain and evidence of increasing abdominal growth. In the final three months there is a faster increase in weight and size before *lightening* and labour occur.

Antenatal care of pregnant women should include a blood test and regular examination by an obstetrician of urine, blood pressure and weight to protect against toxaemia of pregnancy, rhesus factor incompatibility, anaemia, and venereal disease. Abdominal examination should be conducted to ensure that the baby is growing correctly. An obstetrician will also give advice about diet (and extra vitamins and iron that may be required), exercise, rest, special exercises to help in labour, and postnatal care of the baby.

Pregnancy test. A test for pregnancy can be performed on urine that has been collected in a clean bottle. The bottle must not contain any traces of detergents, soap or other chemicals. A pharmacist can perform the test or, with some preparations, the test can be done at home, but it will not be effective until at least ten days after the missed period. Occasionally the result may remain negative, despite repeated tests, even when the woman is pregnant but it is extremely rare for the result to be positive when pregnancy has not occurred.

Premenstrual tension. This may occur during the week preceding a period, particularly as a woman gets older. It is usually

Gynaecological Problems

associated with fluid retention, which gives a feeling of abdominal distension. Symptoms include swollen breasts, weight gain, headaches, and occasionally spots on the face and shoulders. Premenstrual tension may also lead to anxiety and depression.

TREATMENT. Discussion with a doctor may give reassurance that this is a physical and not a psychological illness. Diuretics (fluid-removing drugs) will often help if they are taken for at least a week before the period is due.

Prolapse. A prolapse of the womb (uterus) is caused by a weakening of the muscles and ligaments that hold the womb in its normal position. A prolapsed uterus falls into the vagina pulling the bladder and, to a lesser extent, the bowel with it. The uterine ligaments may have been overstretched in *labour* or weakened after the *menopause*. The indications of a prolapse are not always obvious but there may be a feeling of pressure, as if something has fallen. Involuntary urination when coughing, laughing or lifting something, backache and depression may also be associated with a prolapse.

TREATMENT. An operation to tighten the ligaments is usual but in the elderly a plastic ring can be put in the upper end of the vagina to hold the uterus in place.

Quickening. The first time a pregnant woman feels her baby move is known as "quickening". It is usually a slight fluttering sensation and is normally felt between the 16th and 20th weeks of pregnancy.

Salpingitis. An inflammation of the ducts (Fallopian tubes) from the ovaries to the uterus. The infecting organisms usually spread from the neck of the womb (cervix) through the womb itself to the Fallopian tubes. The causes include infections of the vagina (vaginitis) or the cervix, venereal disease or infection following an *abortion* or *miscarriage*. The symptoms may be acute, with fever, abdominal pain and *vaginal discharge*, or chronic, with dull, lower abdominal pain.

TREATMENT. A doctor must be consulted. Acute cases require admission to hospital where the disease is treated with antibiotics and sometimes an operation to drain an abscess. Chronic salpingitis also needs a long course of antibiotics. Complications of salpingitis may be serious and include peritonitis and sterility.

Smear test (Papanicolaou smear). In the course of a normal vaginal examination a few cells are removed from the surface of the cervix of the womb, so that they can be examined under a microscope. This examination detects whether they are normal, or whether they show signs of infection, abnormalities not due to cancer, or changes that may be early indications of cancer. If the test is performed about once a year, precancerous cells can be detected and highly effective treatment can be given before cancer develops.

Stillbirth. A baby that is born dead after the 28th week of pregnancy is described as stillborn. Death may be caused by congenital abnormalities, prolonged and difficult *labour*, or maternal illness such as high blood pressure or untreated syphilis. An unusually premature birth may cause a baby to be stillborn, but antenatal care reduces the chances of this happening.

Vaginal discharge. The normal vaginal secretion varies within the menstrual cycle, increasing at the time of ovulation and increasing again before and just after menstruation. The amount of discharge varies greatly from woman to woman and is often increased by sexual stimulation, the contraceptive pill, or anxiety. An abnormal discharge, usually indicated by irritation, slight bleeding or unpleasant smell, may be a sign of cervical or uterine infections.

Vaginitis. An infection of the vagina. It may be a mild catarrhal type of infection caused by a variety of organisms including the fungus causing moniliasis (thrush). Vaginitis may also be associated with pregnancy or with the use of the contraceptive pill. It may also occur in diabetes, or as a result of using antibiotics or corticosteroid drugs, or from douching with chemicals that are too strong. Trichomoniasis is a form of vaginitis caused by minute moving parasites that may live in the vagina. Symptoms are not always obvious but they usually cause discharge when the vaginal wall is disturbed by sexual intercourse, menstruation or an illness. Trichomoniasis and moniliasis may also cause the vulva to itch and to discharge profusely, sometimes with slight bleeding.

TREATMENT. The condition must be reported to a doctor for the correct diagnosis to be made. Drugs are usually given in the form of pessaries or creams to put in the vagina. Trichomoniasis also responds to drugs taken by mouth. In trichomoniasis and moniliasis both sexual partners should be treated.

Vulvitis. An inflammation of the vulva, the outer part of the female genitals at the entrance to the vagina. It may be associated with *vaginitis*, herpes infections, an infection of lubricating glands causing abscesses (Bartholin's abscess), or with rubbing from pads or clothes that are too tight.

TREATMENT. Consult a doctor. If the area is very sore and uncomfortable a cold compress will often relieve the symptoms. If the inflammation is painful, drugs such as aspirin may be used until further treatment is started.

Infectious Illnesses

Immunization provides protection against disease. The more common diseases against which protection may be obtained are listed below, together with recommendations for immunization. Each of the diseases mentioned is also described in a separate article in this section.

Cholera. Two injections, one to four weeks apart, are required before travelling to places where cholera is endemic. An international certificate takes effect six days after the first injection and lasts for six months. A booster injection may be given within that time. Immunization gives only moderate protection.

Diphtheria. An injection is usually given at the same time as tetanus and whooping cough (pertussis) immunization as triple antigen (DTP), at the ages of five, six and 12 months. A booster injection is required at five years.

German measles (rubella). A single subcutaneous injection may be given at the age of one. Alternatively, girls aged about 11 years may be immunized.

Influenza. Immunization gives about 70% protection for about six months. The specific vaccine varies each year to combat the particular virus prevalent at that time.

Measles. Immunization at the age of 15 months gives 98% protection. The injection may produce mild catarrh, fever and a

Infectious Illnesses

slight rash about ten days later. It will protect against natural infection if it is given within three days of contact.

Mumps. Immunization is not routinely given but can be useful to protect adults who have not had mumps. It will not protect if the patient is already in quarantine.

Poliomyelitis. An oral vaccine is given at the same time as immunization for diphtheria, tetanus and whooping cough. Boosters are required at the ages of five and ten years.

Smallpox. This is not given routinely because the risks of a fatal reaction from the vaccine are greater than the risks of catching the natural disease, which is now almost extinct. An international certificate is required for a few countries. The effect of the first (primary) vaccination must be examined after a week to ensure that it has produced an effect.

Tetanus. Immunization is usually given at the same time as diphtheria and whooping cough immunization (triple antigen). A booster is required at the age of five and then repeated every five years or after a dirty wound or cut.

Tuberculosis. This vaccine, also known as the BCG vaccine, is given at the age of 12 to those who have a negative skin test for tuberculosis. Immunization usually gives life-long protection.

Typhoid. Partial protection is achieved from two injections given two to four weeks apart. A booster is required every two years. The vaccine often causes a feverish reaction and a sore arm for about a day.

Typhus. Two subcutaneous injections are given a week apart. An international certificate may be required.

Whooping cough (pertussis). This is usually given at the same time as diphtheria and tetanus immunization (triple antigen). In rare cases it may cause a severe reaction and this possibility should be discussed with a doctor before starting the injections. It is not advisable for infants who have had fits, or who have a family history of severe allergy or eczema.

Yellow fever. Protection lasts about ten years starting ten days after one injection. An international certificate is required by many countries.

Chickenpox (varicella). Infection by a virus related to Herpes zoster which causes *shingles.* The incubation period may be up to three weeks and the patient is infectious for about two days before the onset of the rash until six days after the rash first appears. A period of three weeks' quarantine is required from the last time of contact. The symptoms include fever followed two or three days later by small red spots on the body which develop into clear blisters, then become milky in colour and form scabs after three or four days. New spots may occur in the next three days and are often preceded by a rise in temperature.

TREATMENT. Treat as for fever. A doctor may recommend antihistamine drugs and calamine lotion. Do not scratch the spots as this can lead to infection of the blisters, causing permanent scars.

Quarantine: 21 days after last contact with the infection.

Cholera. A water-borne bacterial infection that occurs principally in the tropics. The first symptoms appear within five days of contracting the disease. Frequent, watery diarrhoea and a slight fever are accompanied by violent vomiting and abdominal cramps. The greatest, potentially fatal, danger is from dehydration leading to shock and circulatory failure.

94

Infectious Illnesses

TREATMENT. Antibiotics may help to reduce the diarrhoea but intravenous replacement of fluids and salts lost through vomiting and diarrhoea is essential. This must be performed in hospital. Adequate sanitation, hygiene, immunization with a cholera vaccine and avoidance of unboiled water are necessary precautions for protection against cholera.

Quarantine: one week after contact with the disease.

Diphtheria. An acute, highly contagious and often fatal bacterial infection that usually affects the mucous membranes of the throat. The symptoms develop after about two to seven days' incubation, and include severe sore throat, fever, and respiratory obstruction with patches of grey membrane in the throat. The toxin produced by the bacteria may cause heart failure, palpitations, and polyneuritis.

TREATMENT. An artificial opening in the windpipe (tracheostomy) may be required if breathing is very difficult. Treatment with a diphtheria antitoxin and antibiotics is essential, followed by a slow convalescence with the strictest bed rest, particularly if the heart has been affected. The diphtheria membrane should not be interfered with unless it obstructs breathing.

Quarantine: Those who have been in contact with the disease should remain in quarantine until repeated throat cultures are negative.

Dysentery. An inflammation of the digestive tract due to an infection from contaminated food and water. The symptoms include diarrhoea, with blood and mucus, fever and abdominal pain. The infecting organisms may be bacterial or unicellular. Amoebic dysentery is usually found only in tropical countries and may also infect the liver. Bacillary dysentery is caused by Shigella bacteria, and usually develops four or five days after infection.

TREATMENT. The faeces must be examined, and antibiotic treatment follows an exact diagnosis. General care should be as for diarrhoea. The faeces must be examined again after treatment to ensure that the infection has been eliminated.

German measles (rubella). A virus infection that causes a mild fever and sore throat for one or two days, followed by a fine, orange-pink rash on the face and spreads over the body. The rash lasts two or three days. Tender, swollen glands at the back of the head may last for about ten days. Adults with German measles may develop painful swollen joints of the limbs. The most serious complications of rubella affect the child born to a woman who has the disease during the first three months of pregnancy. Cataracts, congenital heart problems, deafness, and other abnormalities may be found in the baby.

TREATMENT. Treat as for fever. Lotions to soothe the itching may help. The patient must be isolated from any woman who might be in the early (undetected) stages of pregnancy or in the first three months of pregnancy.

Quarantine: 21 days after last contact with the disease.

Influenza ('flu). A virus infection that commonly reaches epidemic proportions. The type of virus varies from time to time so that immunity to the disease is difficult to acquire. The incubation period of the disease is about 48 hours. Symptoms include the acute onset of fever, sometimes with vomiting, a temperature up to 104°F (40°C), headache, sore

95

Infectious Illnesses

throat, aching muscles, and often a slight cough. An attack usually lasts about three to six days. Complications include bronchitis, pneumonia, sinusitis, and otitis media.

TREATMENT. Treat as for fever. Rest, good ventilation and isolation from others are recommended. Consult a doctor if the cough increases or the temperature remains high.

Malaria. A tropical illness caused by a unicellular organism (plasmodium) transmitted by the bite of the Anopheles mosquito. Symptoms include intermittent high fever, sometimes with delirium, recurring every few days depending on the type of infection. Malignant malaria causes blockage of the blood vessels, coma, kidney failure and death. Prolonged, recurrent malaria produces anaemia and listlessness.

TREATMENT. Antimalarial drugs are required after careful diagnosis and study by a specialist in tropical medicine. Anyone who develops a fever and who has recently been to a malarious area must consult a doctor at once.

Those intending to visit a malarious region may be protected by regular medication with antimalarial drugs. The drugs should be taken throughout the stay and should be continued for a month after leaving the area. Mosquito netting around the bed is also recommended.

Measles (rubeola). A virus infection, the symptoms of which include fever with catarrh, sore throat and conjunctivitis for three to five days before the onset of a fine, pink-red rash that starts behind the ears and spreads over the face and down to the trunk and limbs. The incubation period may be up to two weeks, but is usually about ten days. Measles is infectious from the onset of fever until five days after the rash appears. For one or two days before the rash, tiny red spots with white centres (Koplik's spots) may be noticed inside the cheeks or on the palate. A dry, unproductive cough, a headache and profound malaise are present throughout the illness. Complications include bronchitis, otitis media, sinusitis, and, rarely, encephalitis.

TREATMENT. Treat as a fever. The patient should be isolated in a well-ventilated room, with the curtains drawn if the eyes are painful. Complications will require a doctor's diagnosis and treatment with antibiotics. Severe cases, and those with encephalitis, need hospital treatment.

Quarantine: two weeks after last contact with the disease.

Meningitis. An inflammation of the membranes surrounding the brain and spinal cord, caused by viral or bacterial infections. Symptoms include a severe headache, fever, intolerance of light, stiff neck, and vomiting. Meningitis may damage the brain and nervous system, and may prove fatal.

TREATMENT. Urgent admission to hospital for investigation and treatment with antibiotics is essential. The patient should be isolated. Darkness and quiet are essential as excitement may cause the patient to have convulsions.

Mononucleosis, infectious (glandular fever). A virus infection spread by close contact. Diagnosis is confirmed by blood tests. Symptoms include malaise, sore throat, fever, enlarged spleen, swollen lymph glands, and general weakness. Diagnosis is confirmed by blood tests. The onset is often sudden, and the infection usually lasts for two or three weeks. The main complication is jaundice.

TREATMENT. Treat as a fever with bed rest during the acute

Infectious Illnesses

stage. A doctor must be consulted and care is necessary when giving antibiotics as the body may react abnormally in the course of this disease. A gradual return to normal life is necessary because over-activity may cause a relapse.

Mumps. A virus infection that causes inflammation and swelling of the parotid and other salivary glands in the mouth and throat. Symptoms develop gradually with headache, slight fever and pain behind the ears leading to marked swelling of the parotid glands beneath the angle of the jaw. The swelling usually lasts for about a week. The most serious complications are inflammation of the testicles in adult males and the breasts and ovaries in women, which may cause sterility. Occasionally mumps may also affect the hearing.

TREATMENT. Treat as a fever, with bed rest, plenty of fluids, and a diet that does not require chewing. Cold compresses may help to control swelling of the testicles. Immunization is also possible.

Quarantine: 28 days from last contact with the disease.

Poliomyelitis. An infection of the spinal cord caused by the water-borne polio virus. The symptoms of the minor form of polio include mild fever, headache, stiff neck and muscle ache, and last for two or three days. In the major form of polio, which is less common, these symptoms are followed by the rapid onset of high fever, muscle pains, intolerance of light and severe headache. The final stage is the weakness or paralysis of some muscles which may limit breathing and sometimes cause death. Only about 10% of those infected with poliomyelitis develop the major form of the illness and not all of these are left paralysed. The symptoms appear about two or three weeks after the victim has caught the disease and it remains infectious for a further three weeks.

TREATMENT. Isolation in hospital with complete rest. Pain-killing drugs and artificial respiration may be needed. Immunization of children is strongly advised and anyone who has been in contact with the disease should be revaccinated.

Rabies (hydrophobia). A disease caused by a virus transmitted in the saliva of an infected warm-blooded animal, usually by a bite. The animals most commonly responsible for transmitting rabies are dogs, foxes and bats. The incubation period is usually about five weeks, but the symptoms may appear as soon as a week or as long as a year after the bite. Symptoms include extreme mental excitement, severe muscle spasms, especially of the throat when drinking, and ultimately respiratory paralysis and death.

TREATMENT. Anti-rabies vaccine must be given as soon as possible after being bitten by an infected animal. There is no effective treatment of the disease once the symptoms appear. Any animal that appears unusually aggressive should be considered a potential carrier of rabies and should be examined for the disease. Vaccination of an animal may protect it from the disease but immunity is not guaranteed and a quarantine period of six months is also required.

Scarlet fever (scarlatina). A contagious infection due to streptococcus bacteria that causes a characteristic scarlet rash. The symptoms develop from one to six days after contact and include sore throat, fever, rapid pulse, rash and inflamed tongue. Peeling skin and thinning hair may also occur.

TREATMENT. Penicillin should be given for at least ten days,

Infectious Illnesses

following a doctor's advice. The patient should be isolated and kept in bed and the symptoms treated as a fever. Antibiotic treatment is necessary to prevent complications such as rheumatic fever or nephritis.

Quarantine: Until throat swabs are negative.

Shingles (Herpes zoster). A virus related to *chickenpox* that affects part of a cranial or spinal nerve and causes painful spots and blisters to erupt along the course of a peripheral nerve. Typically it affects the trunk of the body or the face. Symptoms include local pain, malaise and slight fever followed by red rash over the distribution of the nerve endings, which develops into clear blisters that become milky and then form scabs after three or four days. The pain is variable and may be intense. Complications include eye problems caused by the involvement of a facial nerve, infection of the blisters, and pain in the nerve which may last for several months after the disease has disappeared.

TREATMENT. Consult a doctor. Special anti-herpes solutions can help if treatment with them is started at the onset of the disease. Pain-killing drugs, bed rest, a light, nutritious diet and adequate convalescence are usually required.

Smallpox (variola). An acute contagious virus infection characterized by the appearance of pustules. The disease has an incubation period of one or two weeks and remains infectious until all scabs have disappeared. Smallpox is indicated by the sudden onset of high fever with severe illness. On the third day a rash of spots and blisters appears on the arms and legs and spreads to the trunk. The scabs separate during the next two or three weeks, leaving pitted scars.

TREATMENT. Isolation in hospital with skilled nursing care is essential. Plenty of water, fruit and vegetables are recommended. Particular care must be taken with the eyes, which should be bathed regularly.

Quarantine: A period of two weeks from the time of contact, with vaccination or revaccination as soon as possible.

Tetanus (lockjaw). Disease marked by painful spasms of the muscles of the jaw or other parts of the body. They are caused by the tetanus bacillus, which grows at the site of a wound and produces a toxin that causes the muscles to move with reflex spasms. These symptoms develop several days or weeks after the wound has become infected. The spasms are exhausting and, if they affect the respiratory muscles, may cause asphyxia. They are usually associated with fever and the disease is often fatal.

TREATMENT. Proper medical attention must be given to dirty wounds. Anti-tetanus serum and antibiotics are required to prevent the development of the disease. Immunization is recommended and a booster is required from time to time.

Tuberculosis. A bacterial infection, caused by bacteria of the Mycobacterium genus, that may affect the respiratory system, gastrointestinal and urogenital tracts, the nervous system, joints and bones or the skin. The disease may be carried by people, cattle or birds. Tuberculosis develops gradually, causing symptoms of malaise, fever, loss of weight and often a cough. The infection may also remain dormant for long periods, causing the symptoms to recur from time to time as the disease progresses.

TREATMENT. Drugs are effective in most cases but treatment

may have to continue for up to two years. Contacts require chest X-rays and BCG vaccination. Immunization protects those who have not been in contact with the disease.

Typhoid (enteric fever). An infection, due to bacteria of the Salmonella genus, that is spread by contaminated water, milk and food. Symptoms include the gradual onset of fever, headache, constipation, cough, and scattered pink spots on the trunk, and usually appear within three weeks of contracting the disease. Complications include intestinal haemorrhage and perforation of the bowel causing peritonitis.

TREATMENT. Isolation in hospital is required for treatment with antibiotics. Examination of the faeces is necessary to ensure that the disease has been cured.

Typhus. A group of diseases carried by lice, ticks and fleas. Symptoms appear abruptly a few days to three weeks after being bitten. There is usually a large red scab at the site of the bite. This is followed by a high fever, severe headache, delirium, the appearance of purple spots on the trunk and limbs, and severe illness lasting for seven to ten days.

TREATMENT. The most common form of typhus is associated with unhygienic conditions and may be prevented by adequate sanitation and cleanliness. Immunization is temporarily effective. Hospital treatment with antibiotics is required

Whooping cough (pertussis). A bacterial infection, particularly dangerous to children. The incubation period is usually about ten days and the disease is infectious for about three weeks. Symptoms include catarrh with mild fever at the onset followed by a cough that increases in severity. The cough starts with a spasm and ends with a sharp intake of breath, the whoop. A prolonged coughing spell is often followed by vomiting. Whooping cough may last up to five or six weeks and may cause nose-bleeds, debility and insomnia. Complications include encephalitis and pneumonia.

TREATMENT. Antibiotics given in the early stages may help. No effective cough mixture is available. Bed rest, sedation at night, sufficient fluid to drink and frequent light meals help to sustain the patient through the course of the disease. Patients should be observed carefully for complications.

Quarantine: 21 days after last contact with the disease.

Yellow fever. A virus infection carried by mosquitoes. It occurs particularly in central Africa and parts of South America. The symptoms of fever, vomiting, dehydration, muscle pains and jaundice appear within a week of being bitten.

TREATMENT. Immunization provides protection in areas where yellow fever is endemic. There is no specific treatment for those who suffer from the disease, but rest, fluid replacement and a nutritious, liquid diet, supplemented with vitamin K and calcium gluconate, help to sustain the patient through the course of the illness.

Joint and Bone Problems

Ankylosis. Ankylosis is the stiffening or fixation of a joint due to disease or injury. The more extreme "bony" (or "true") ankylosis is the fusion of the two bones that form the joint. Spondylosis is a general term for ankylosis of a vertebral joint or degenerative changes in the spine due to *arthritis*. Spondylitis specifically refers to inflammation of the vertebrae, and ankylosing spondylitis is arthritis of the spine.

Joint and Bone Problems

Arthritis. An inflammation of a joint. There are several distinct arthritic disorders. Osteoarthritis is the degeneration of a joint's surface due to age or to excessive use. Rheumatoid arthritis is a general disease of several joints marked by inflammation of the membranes and joint surfaces. The symptoms are increasing pain, swelling and disability over a number of years.

TREATMENT. Various anti-rheumatic drugs can be used but aspirin in regular doses is the most helpful. Relief can be gained from regular muscle exercises and injections of corticosteroid drugs, although the latter may have serious side-effects. Devices to help the arthritic include special shoes for deformed feet and mechanical aids to help with dressing, washing and eating. Operations on the joints and, in some cases, joint replacement surgery may be required.

Bursitis. Bursae are found at parts of the body where friction may occur, such as in the knee and elbow joints. They are pouch-like cavities lined with synovial membrane and filled with synovial fluid. Inflammation of a bursa is called bursitis and should be treated as *capsulitis* or *synovitis*. Housemaid's knee and tennis elbow are common examples of bursitis.

Capsulitis. Inflammation of the fibrous tissue that encloses a synovial joint, particularly the shoulder joint. Capsulitis is usually caused by a strain or injury, and is indicated by pain and restriction of movement.

TREATMENT. The affected joint must be rested. Aspirin and anti-rheumatic drugs or possibly an injection of corticosteroid drugs into the capsule may be required.

Cartilage, torn. An injury to the cartilage of the knee. Each knee has two thin, crescent-shaped pieces of cartilage which assist normal movement of the joint. A sudden twist or injury to the knee may tear the cartilage, causing sharp pain. The knee locks in one position or gives way.

TREATMENT. A large firm crepe bandage should be bound round the straightened knee. Pain-killing drugs are usually required. If symptoms continue, surgical removal of the cartilage may be necessary.

Dislocation. A painful injury to a joint in which one or both surfaces are forced out of their normal position. Subluxation describes a partial or incomplete dislocation. The joint is unable to move and there may be obvious deformity. The casualty should be treated initially as if the joint were fractured and should be taken to hospital as soon as possible.

Fracture. General term for a broken bone. A fracture is described as being simple if the bone is broken cleanly with no external wound, and greenstick if only one side of the bone is cracked and the other side is bent. In a compound or open fracture the external wound extends to the fracture. A fracture is called comminuted if the bone is broken in more than one place. In a complicated fracture the bone damages nearby structures such as a nerve, artery or organ, and in an impacted one the bone ends are jammed together. A stress fracture is due to repeated minor injury, as may occur in a foot when running on hard ground and a pathological fracture is due to a disease, such as cancer, that has weakened the bone. For treatment of fractures, see FIRST AID TECHNIQUES, pp.25-29.

Frozen shoulder. This describes a painful shoulder, the movement of which is restricted. It may be associated with fib-

Mouth and Throat Problems

rositis, *bursitis*, *capsulitis*, or sometimes with a heart attack or chest problem. Recovery may take a long time.

TREATMENT. Pain-killing and anti-rheumatic drugs, shortwave heat treatment and physiotherapy may help and an injection of corticosteroid drugs is sometimes effective.

Gout. A disorder of the body's metabolism (hyperuricaemia) in which the normal disposal of uric acid is disrupted. As a result, salts of uric acid accumulate in the joints causing pain and inflammation. Ultimately gout may cause *arthritis* of the affected joints. It may also involve the kidneys where crystallized uric acid may be deposited. Attacks may be precipitated by a large meal, drinking alcohol, illness, an operation, an accident, or fatigue.

TREATMENT. An acute attack can be treated under medical supervision with large doses of anti-rheumatic drugs. Anti-gout drugs will help to prevent attacks by reducing the level of uric acid in the body. The pain is eased by rest with the affected joints raised. Massage and warmth from hot dressings may also give relief.

Rickets (rachitis). A disease, caused by vitamin D deficiency that causes softening and subsequently deformity of the bones, particularly in children. The most obvious deformities are distorted spine, knock-knees, bow legs, and pigeon chest. A deficiency of vitamin D in adults will cause calcium to be lost from the bones, leading to osteomalacia.

TREATMENT. As a deficiency disease, rickets can be prevented by sunshine and a balanced diet that provides an adequate intake of vitamin D.

Synovitis. An inflammation or infection of the membranes that produce synovial fluid. These membranes and their synovial fluid surround tendons, joints, and other places where friction occurs. Inflammation of these places may also be described as tendinitis, *capsulitis* or *bursitis*, and occurs because of injuries or strains, infections, or diseases such as rheumatoid *arthritis*. Symptoms include pain, local tenderness and swelling, and difficulties in movement.

TREATMENT. The affected joint or limb should be rested, using a sling or splint if necessary. Antibiotics, aspirin, anti-rheumatic drugs, or injection of corticosteroid drugs may be required, following a doctor's advice.

Water on the knee. A knee swollen by excess fluid in the joint cavity under the knee-cap. It may be caused by an injury to the knee, a torn *cartilage*, *arthritis* or *synovitis*.

TREATMENT. Tie a firm crepe bandage around the knee when it is straight and rest the knee as much as possible. Aspirin and anti-rheumatic drugs sometimes help. If the symptoms persist exercises are necessary to keep thigh muscles strong. In all cases a doctor should be consulted.

Mouth and Throat Problems

Bad breath (halitosis). This may be caused by smoking, by infections of the nose, gums, mouth or lungs, tooth decay, certain foods, fasting, stomach disorders, constipation or by general disease. Smoking is probably the commonest cause.

TREATMENT. The cause should be treated. Stop smoking, treat local mouth infections, clean the teeth regularly, and try to eat a light, easily digestible diet. Consult a doctor or dentist if the condition persists.

Mouth and Throat Problems

Cold sore. Recurrent blisters that break and form sores around the lips, often associated with a cold or fever. They are caused by a virus (Herpes simplex) that lives in the body and causes symptoms only when resistance is lowered.

TREATMENT. Immediate application of an anti-viral preparation may be effective. Various proprietary lotions or tincture of benzoin compound (Friar's balsam) may also help.

Gingivitis. An inflammation of the gums that starts around the teeth. The gums become swollen and tender and are likely to bleed. If it is not treated an infection around the teeth (periodontitis) may occur.

TREATMENT. Regular brushing of the teeth and a diet of food that needs chewing, without sugar and with plenty of vitamins, helps to prevent inflammation. Dental treatment of decayed teeth and regular scraping of tartar from the enamel is also necessary.

Glossitis. This inflammation results in a smooth, red, sometimes sore tongue. It may be due to the excessive use of antibiotics or other medicaments, or to a lack of vitamins of the B group. It may also be a symptom of pernicious anaemia.

TREATMENT. Extra vitamin B should be given, and antiseptic mouth washes used sparingly. A doctor should be consulted if there is no improvement after a few days.

Gumboil. An abscess on the gum, usually caused by infection of a decayed tooth.

TREATMENT. Pain-killing drugs, antiseptic mouth washes and gargles help until the gumboil can be seen by a dentist or a doctor. Treatment with antibiotics may be required before the tooth decay can be dealt with.

Moniliasis (thrush). An infection of the skin or mucous membranes of the mouth and throat, due to the fungus Monilia (Candida) albicans. It affects babies and young children in particular. The symptoms of white patches and ulcers in the mouth and at the top of the throat are often associated with gastrointestinal problems and fever. See also *Skin Problems: Moniliasis*; *Urogenital Problems: Moniliasis*.

TREATMENT. Consult a doctor for advice about the appropriate antifungal drugs or preparations.

Strep throat. An infection of the throat by a strain of streptococcus bacteria. The symptoms include marked inflammation, pain on swallowing, and fever. Infections of this type spread easily and if left untreated may lead to serious infections elsewhere in the body. See also *Tonsillitis*.

TREATMENT. Consult a doctor as soon as possible. Antibiotic therapy is usually required. To gargle with antiseptic mouth wash may relieve the inflammation.

Throat, sore. A sore throat can occur with any infection of the respiratory tract. It may also be caused by smoking or by breathing in a smoky atmosphere. If the soreness persists for more than 12 hours, if it becomes worse, or if it is associated with fever, it may be a symptom of influenza, *tonsillitis*, mononucleosis, or a throat infection caused by a virus or by bacteria such as streptococci (see *Strep throat*). Throat infections are easily transmitted, and a persistent sore throat should be reported to a doctor.

TREATMENT. When the soreness is first noticed, gargle with soluble aspirin in warm water and swallow. Avoid crowded places so that the disease does not spread.

Muscle and Tendon Problems

Tonsillitis. An inflammation due to infection of the lymphatic tissue at the back of the mouth (tonsils). With the adenoids in the nose the tonsils protect the throat and lungs from infecting organisms that may enter through the mouth and nose. They help to establish immunity to common infective agents and are most active in childhood, when many infections are encountered for the first time. Large tonsils are not abnormal at this age. If the tonsils are no longer able to cope with infections they may become inflamed and tonsillitis will occur. The symptoms of this are a sore throat, a fever, and persistent malaise. Recurrent attacks of tonsillitis, or a chronic infection lasting several years, may be indications for their removal (tonsillectomy).

TREATMENT. A doctor must be consulted. Gargle with soluble aspirin in warm water, and swallow it. Antiseptic mouth washes and throat lozenges also help. In more serious cases the doctor may use antibiotics to combat the infection.

Toothache. Pain in or around a tooth, which may be so severe that it appears to affect the whole side of the jaw. It may be caused by an infection in the tooth itself due to food that has lodged in a cavity or it may be due to a *gumboil* around the base of the tooth. In children toothache may be caused by a secondary tooth pushing at the root of a milk tooth that is due to fall.

TREATMENT. Dental treatment is required in most cases, and medical advice may also be required for treatment of a gumboil. Toothache is most easily prevented by dental care in the home and by regular visits to a dentist.

Ulcer, mouth. A small blister that commonly occurs on the side or tip of the tongue and ruptures to form a small painful spot. The ulcer is usually white with an inflamed rim. Ulcers may occur because of indigestion, anxiety, irritation of the tongue by the rough surface of a tooth, or because of a cold.

TREATMENT. A mouth wash reduces the inflammation and ulcers normally heal rapidly without further treatment. If necessary a proprietary ointment may be used.

Muscle and Tendon Problems

Achilles' tendon. The tendon from the heel to the muscle of the calf. This may rupture, particularly in the middle-aged, because of sudden strain on it when running or jumping. When this occurs there is a severe pain at the back of the ankle, accompanied by an inability to stand on tip toe.

TREATMENT. An operation is required to repair the tendon. In certain cases the injury is allowed to heal in plaster of Paris without an operation but this risks leaving the patient with a permanently weak ankle.

Calf pain on walking. If this occurs regularly after mild exercise, such as walking, it is a symptom of poor blood supply. It may be due to anaemia but is more commonly a symptom of arteriosclerosis. If it occurs suddenly a doctor should be consulted as soon as possible. It may indicate a pulled muscle or, more seriously, a deep venous thrombosis.

TREATMENT. Consult a doctor for advice. If arteriosclerosis is the cause, stop smoking, reduce weight and avoid eating animal fats. A doctor may recommend drugs to dilate the blood vessels. Sometimes an operation is required to replace a diseased segment of artery.

Muscle and Tendon Problems

Carpal tunnel syndrome. This is caused by the swelling of a ligament which presses on a nerve in the carpal tunnel of the wrist. The symptoms include tingling and sometimes weakness in the index and middle fingers and the thumb. The patient is liable to wake at night from the pain, which is aggravated by excessive use of the wrist. The syndrome is sometimes associated with premenstrual tension.

TREATMENT. Splinting the wrist and injections of corticosteroid drugs may help. An operation may be necessary to divide the ligament and so remove the pressure on the nerve.

Cramp. A painful muscular spasm. This temporary spasm may be caused by a poor blood supply due to cold or a disease such as arteriosclerosis. Cramp may also be caused by insufficient salt in the diet to replace that lost by sweating, or by repetitive movements, as in writer's cramp.

TREATMENT. Warm, rub and stretch the cramped muscle. Increase the dietary intake of salt. Consult a doctor if the cramp persists.

Fibrositis. Inflammation of fibrous connective tissue most commonly associated with stiff and aching shoulders and back. It may be caused by over-exercise or by cold. See also *Rheumatism*.

Neck, stiff. This may be a symptom of muscle strain, but if it persists it may indicate *rheumatism*, *fibrositis*, or possibly a slipped disc.

TREATMENT. Warmth on the affected area and massage may relieve the stiffness. If it persists, consult a doctor.

Rheumatism. A general term used to describe persistent aches in the muscles and joints due to inflammation or other disorders of connective tissue, and frequently associated with cold and damp weather. It is not recognized as a specific disease but may be a symptom of many.

TREATMENT. The disorder that causes the symptoms of rheumatism should be diagnosed and treated. The symptoms may be alleviated by warmth and by drugs such as aspirin.

Sprain. An injury to the ligaments around a joint, caused by a violent, sudden movement. It usually affects the ankle or the wrist. The symptoms are pain, swelling and an inability to move the joint.

TREATMENT. Treat as a fracture until the injury has been examined by a doctor.

Tendinitis. Inflammation of a tendon. It resembles bursitis and synovitis, which are discussed in *Joint and Bone Problems*.

Tenosynovitis. Inflammation of the sheath of a tendon, causing swelling and pain when the tendon is moved. In certain cases a grating sensation accompanies movement.

TREATMENT. The inflammation will usually disappear with rest, but in severe cases it may be necessary to drain the fluid from the tendon sheath. Treatment with anti-rheumatic and corticosteroid drugs is sometimes necessary.

Nervous System Disorders

Bell's palsy. An inflammation of the facial nerve. It causes paralysis of the muscles of facial expression in particular and typically affects only one side of the face, causing the mouth and the eyelids to droop. The inflammation may be painful.

TREATMENT. Analgesics relieve any pain. Recovery is usually complete in a few weeks and may be helped by the use of

Nervous System Disorders

corticosteroid drugs. In rare cases that do not improve, an operation may be necessary.

Concussion. This term commonly refers to concussion of the brain, caused by a jarring blow to the head. It is often associated with temporary loss of consciousness, and vomiting may occur as consciousness returns. Headache, lack of concentration, irritability, and loss of memory may accompany the process of recovery.

TREATMENT. Treat as for shock initially — see the FIRST AID section, p.13. Rest until all the symptoms have disappeared, with bed rest for the first 24 hours. It is important to avoid drinking alcohol.

Convulsions and fits. Seizures characterized by violent muscular spasms that are frequently brief and recurrent. A convulsion may be long-lasting and violent or it may appear as little more than fainting accompanied by slight twitching. Convulsions may be a symptom of *epilepsy*, certain forms of poisoning, malnutrition, or of an illness such as meningitis or tetanus that affects the central nervous system.

TREATMENT. The victim must be protected from injury against hard objects. Make sure that the breathing is not obstructed. When the fit has passed, leave the victim facedown with the head on one side, in the recovery position (see the FIRST AID section, p. 12). As soon as possible, call for medical advice. Cool a child if there is fever because this may have caused the fit.

Epilepsy. Periodic and uncontrollable moments of confusion, loss of attention or unconsciousness. These may be accompanied by fainting or, in more severe cases, by convulsions. The cause of epilepsy is often not known.

Epilepsy is classified in two forms, known as petit mal and grand mal. Petit mal describes momentary loss of awareness lasting about a second. It is more common in children and attacks tend to diminish in frequency and severity with age. Grand mal attacks are typically preceded by strange sensations of smell, taste, and touch. The attack itself involves loss of consciousness and a stiffening of the limbs which lasts about 30 seconds. This is followed by rhythmical muscle contractions, often incontinence of urine, and sometimes guttural noises lasting for about a minute. The victim then lies unconscious, breathing heavily, for a few minutes before recovering sufficiently to move. Confusion and a severe headache may follow an attack, but these symptoms are not always noticed as the victim commonly falls into a deep sleep. Status epilepticus occurs when one grand mal fit continues into another.

TREATMENT. For treatment during an attack, see *Convulsions and fits*. A person who suffers from epilepsy must be examined thoroughly by a doctor. Many anti-epileptic drugs are available and most epileptics lead normal lives, despite restrictions against driving and against working with dangerous machinery or at unusual heights. A regular way of life and a diet that avoids alcohol are recommended.

Multiple sclerosis. A chronic disease of the nervous system. It develops over many years during which time increasingly severe attacks alternate with apparent recovery. Symptoms include double vision, weakness, local numbness, dizziness, difficulty in speaking, increasing *paralysis* and blindness.

Nervous System Disorders

The cause of the disease is not known, although it rarely starts in people more than 40 years old.

TREATMENT. Corticosteroid drugs may ease individual attacks. Practical advice may be obtained from charitable associations that exist to help victims of multiple sclerosis and to promote research.

Paralysis. Loss of strength in a muscle or group of muscles. It is indicated by obvious disability and also by impairment of specific functions such as blinking, speech, urination or use of a limb. Paralysis is usually due to damage to the nervous system caused by a disease such as *polyneuritis* or poliomyelitis, by a *stroke* or by an injury. It may also be psychological in origin and if no other symptoms appear this possibility should be investigated.

TREATMENT. The cause must be determined, usually by hospital investigation. During recovery it is important to keep the muscles active, and treatment and advice from a physiotherapist are necessary.

Parkinson's disease. A nervous disease characterized by trembling and muscular weakness. It usually develops gradually from a slight trembling of the hands over several years to generalized muscular debility. The disease, most common in the elderly, does not affect the intellect.

TREATMENT. Anti-Parkinsonian drugs, particularly Levodopa, are usually effective but in severe cases brain surgery may be required. It is important to treat chest and respiratory disorders at once to prevent complications developing.

Polyneuritis. An inflammation of more than one nerve. Symptoms include numbness, tingling, muscle pain, double vision, weakness and *paralysis*, and may be due to poisoning by lead, insecticides or other chemicals, to diabetes, vitamin B deficiency, infections such as diphtheria or mumps, or to cancer, often cancer of the lung.

TREATMENT. The cause must be determined, and if the symptoms are severe, treated in hospital. Physiotherapy and vitamin B supplements may assist recovery.

Stroke. A circulatory problem affecting the brain and causing symptoms elsewhere in the body. The brain is damaged because the blood supply to a part of it is cut off by the blockage or deterioration of a cerebral artery. The symptoms indicate which part of the brain has been damaged. A stroke may cause momentary weakness, numbness, disordered speech, or double vision, which may be followed by complete recovery. A serious stroke may result in paralysis of half the body (hemiplegia) or death.

TREATMENT. Call a doctor or an ambulance immediately. Do not give the patient anything to drink. Lay the patient facedown with the head to one side in the recovery position and observe carefully that heart and breathing do not stop.

Nose Problems

Adenoids. Pads of lymphatic tissue at the back of the nasal passages. Infection causes them to swell, leading to symptoms such as catarrh and *snoring* and to secondary disorders such as middle ear infections and deafness.

TREATMENT. Nose drops, antihistamines or antibiotics may be prescribed. Recurrent infections benefit from the surgical removal of the adenoids (adenoidectomy).

Psychiatric Problems

Hay fever (allergic rhinitis). An allergy affecting the mucous air passages of the nose and throat. It is caused by grass or flower pollens, hay or house dust, and other external irritants. Pollen allergies are seasonal and tend to occur at the same time each year for the individual sufferer. Symptoms include catarrhal inflammation, a running nose, sneezing and watering eyes. Asthmatic symptoms may also occur.

TREATMENT. Inoculations with extracts of the particular allergen are sometimes successful. Antihistamines reduce symptoms but introduce problems, such as drowsiness, which may be unacceptable, especially at work or when driving. Anti-inflammatory nasal sprays control the symptoms in most patients.

Nose-bleed (epistaxis). Haemorrhage from the nose may be caused by colds, catarrh, blowing the nose too hard, injury, foreign bodies in the nasal passage or changes in atmospheric pressure. It may also be associated with arteriosclerosis, violent exertion, bleeding disorders or with the hormonal changes of puberty and menstruation.

TREATMENT. Sit quietly, with the head supported, leaning forward over a bowl, and apply cold compresses to the nose or the back of the neck. Avoid breathing through the nose. A severe nose-bleed may be treated medically with adrenalin.

Sinusitis. Inflammation of the accessory nasal cavities which open into the main nasal passages. Symptoms are variable pain over the affected sinus, catarrh and possibly fever. Causes include allergies, colds, catarrh, measles, tooth infection and diving. Some people are predisposed to sinusitis because of inadequate drainage of the sinuses, which may be caused by a deviated nasal septum or by chronic rhinitis.

TREATMENT. Consult a doctor. Nose drops, steam inhalations, antihistamines, pain-killing drugs or antibiotics may be recommended.

Snoring. Noisy breathing while asleep. It may be caused by catarrh, enlarged *adenoids* or a deviated nasal septum. For most people, however, it is simply the result of sleeping on the back with the mouth open which causes vibration of the back of the palate.

Psychiatric Problems

Alcoholism. The compulsive need for alcohol. Some people who depend on alcohol drink steadily and others have occasional heavy drinking bouts that continue for several days. Symptoms that indicate alcoholism include increasing inefficiency, aggressiveness, polyneuritis, and the deterioration of personal and family relationships. Further complications include vitamin deficiency, cirrhosis of the liver, gastritis, seizures and *delirium tremens*.

TREATMENT. Treatment is effective only when the patient really wants to be cured. A "drying out" period is required with sedation to avoid the hazards of delirium tremens. Continued help from a psychiatrist or from Alcoholics Anonymous may help to maintain stability.

Anorexia nervosa. A loss of appetite for food that cannot be explained by any physical disease but is attributed to *depression*. It is most common in teenage girls. The symptoms include loss of weight, sometimes vomiting after a meal, and often the cessation of periods (amenorrhoea). A person suf-

Psychiatric Problems

fering from anorexia nervosa remains cheerful and active and usually denies that there is any problem.

TREATMENT. Skilled medical advice and often hospital admission are required. Antidepressant and tranquillizing drugs may help, but treatment takes a long time and requires the co-operation of the family as well as the patient.

Anxiety. A common state of mind, often associated with a realistic assessment of difficulties, that may lead to physical symptoms such as sweating, palpitations, trembling, *insomnia*, lassitude, loss of weight and irritability. If a person suffers from *depression*, problems will seem greater and more difficult to cope with and so the anxiety will increase. Sometimes the symptoms of anxiety hide those of depression.

TREATMENT. This may be difficult if the anxiety has a rational basis. It may help to use tranquillizers during the day and mild sedatives at night for a short time but reassurance and moral support are of greater value than drugs. Specific therapy is likely to be most useful if anxiety is associated with depression. If antidepressant drugs remove the symptoms of depression, the problems causing the anxiety may appear less serious.

Autism. A condition in which a person is totally absorbed in subjective thoughts that exclude and are not affected by the external world. In early childhood this failure in mental development prevents normal learning although it does not indicate low intelligence.

TREATMENT. This is difficult and only rarely successful.

Delirium. A condition in which the mental state is disturbed. It may be caused by medicinal or addictive drugs, by high fever, or by infectious illnesses such as typhoid or encephalitis. Typical symptoms include excitement, thought disturbance, confusion and *insomnia*.

TREATMENT. Consult a doctor urgently. The correct treatment of the cause will shorten the illness.

Delirium tremens. A condition that occurs in *alcoholism*. It usually develops when the craving for alcohol is not satisfied and withdrawal symptoms set in. Hallucinations, sudden fears, muscle twitching, insomnia, periods of physical activity, and palpitations affect the patient for several days. Barbiturate addiction may also lead to delirium tremens.

TREATMENT. Admission to hospital for sedation and vitamin B injections is necessary. Recovery is gradual but usually complete after a long convalescence.

Depression. A sense of hopelessness and exhaustion that may follow any illness or treatment, or may occur without obvious cause. It may also be a result of grief or prolonged *anxiety*. Occasionally depression may be associated with periods of high excitement (mania) and it may be a symptom of *manic-depressive illness*. Typical symptoms of depression are lack of concentration, difficulty in making decisions, irritability, pessimism, undue fatigue, *insomnia*, headaches, anxiety, loss of sex drive, tearfulness, suicidal thoughts and sometimes attempted suicide.

TREATMENT. Talking to a doctor about your problems is particularly important, because professional advice is usually the most valuable. Treatment with antidepressant drugs is common and admission to hospital is sometimes necessary for severe cases that require psychiatric help.

Psychiatric Problems

Drug abuse. The compulsive use of drugs due to a physical dependence on their effects and a psychological need for their continued use. The outlines of treatment for the main types of drug abuse are given below, but it should be remembered that each addict requires individual psychiatric assessment and medical care.

Stimulants. The most common stimulants are the amphetamines, cocaine, and others derived from these which are sometimes used alone and sometimes with other drugs such as barbiturates. Stimulants may be taken by mouth, sniffed or injected intravenously. Their effect is to cause a sudden increase of mental or physical activity, euphoria and loss of appetite. This usually leads to a confused mental state which may be accompanied by *paranoia*. Eventually there follows a deep sleep, followed by a period of physical lassitude and *depression*. A serious complication of sniffing cocaine is that this may cause perforation of the nasal membranes. Sedative drugs are required to treat stimulant abuse, together with hospital care, followed by psychiatric assessment and therapy.

Depressants. The most common depressants include alcohol and barbiturates. Depressants are usually taken orally but are also sometimes injected intravenously. Mental confusion, slurred speech and unsteady walking are common effects. Withdrawal symptoms include *anxiety*, *insomnia*, *delirium*, tremor, *delirium tremens* and fits. Hospital admission is required, to treat depressant abuse, followed by psychiatric care.

Opiates. The most common opiates are heroin, morphine and opium. They are sometimes inhaled but heroin and morphine are usually injected intravenously for rapid effect. First experiences produce nausea, vomiting and anxiety. Subsequent doses lead to a state of relaxation and contentment. Tolerance soon develops so that larger doses are required. Withdrawal can be acute with anxiety, irritability, sweating, sneezing, abdominal pain, vomiting, and occasionally fits. Admission to a special drug addiction unit is required to treat opiate addiction, so that sedative drugs and sometimes substitute drugs, such as methadone, can be used to relieve withdrawal symptoms.

Cannabis. The most common forms of cannabis are marijuana (leaves) and hashish (resin), prepared from the leaves and flowers of Cannabis sativa. Dried leaves may be smoked or the resin from the leaves used as an additive to tobacco or to food. Addiction is rare and is psychological rather than physical. The drug causes a mild drowsy state with an increased awareness of colour, sound and taste together with complex mood changes. Chronic users become apathetic, lethargic and have difficulty in concentrating. Certain cases may benefit from psychiatric treatment.

Psychedelics. The most common psychedelics are LSD and mescaline. They promote an increased sense of perception, with images that fluctuate and change in apparently understandable sequences. The effect usually lasts about 12 hours. Occasionally the experience can resemble a nightmare, and sometimes a psychotic or depressed state can result. Acute panic reactions or momentary recurrences of hallucinations may occur during the following few days, and

Psychiatric Problems

these are likely to be the most dangerous aspect of the experience. An individual on a psychedelic "trip" should be accompanied to prevent physical harm. Occasionally admission to hospital is required.

Miscellaneous. A variety of other substances are inhaled or sniffed for the physical or mental experience they give. These include amyl nitrite (a heart drug), nitrous oxide (laughing gas) and some organic solvents used in glues and nail varnishes. Such substances may have serious physiological side-effects.

Hypochondria. An abnormal anxiety about one's health. It may involve imagined illness accompanied by actual pain, and may be associated with *anxiety* or *depression*. It may also indicate personal insecurity that requires repeated reassurance from the authority of a doctor.

Hysteria. A mental state in which the conscious mind is unaware of the real reason for certain thoughts or actions. Hysteria is also regarded as a violent expression of emotion, usually tearful, but this is not the psychiatric use of the term and such emotional outbursts are rarely pathological. In the psychiatric sense, the hysterical patient is genuinely unaware that the pain or illness is imaginary, even though there is no medical evidence to support the complaint.

Insomnia. An inability to sleep. Individuals need different amounts of sleep. Adult requirements vary between four and nine hours every night, babies sleep most of the day, and young children require up to 12 hours a night. Many people wake several times at night and, provided they are not beset by worries, fall asleep again. Insomnia is usually caused by *anxiety, depression*, pain, cold, fever, indigestion, stimulants (such as coffee), or drugs.

TREATMENT. A warm milk drink late in the evening and reading a book in bed sometimes help. Avoid sleeping pills, if possible, as they may perpetuate the need to take them. If insomnia persists for more than a few nights, or if health is affected, consult a doctor.

Mania. A state of nervous excitement associated with an abnormally selfish motivation. Over-enthusiasm, extreme talkativeness, lack of normal inhibitions, failure to maintain a consistent course of action, intolerance of others and a supreme feeling of righteousness are typical symptoms. These are often accompanied by great physical activity and an increased sex drive.

TREATMENT. Sedative drugs and skilled psychiatric care are required. Sometimes compulsory hospital treatment is necessary to prevent megalomania.

Manic-depressive illness. An abnormal mental state characterized by periods of *mania* and severe *depression*. The intensity of the attacks may vary and they are usually separated by periods of relative stability. The illness should not be confused with the normal fluctuations of mood which are a characteristic feature of adolescence.

TREATMENT. The instability of the manic-depressive may be controlled with drugs, but a careful diagnosis by a doctor or psychiatrist is required before any treatment is initiated.

Neurosis. A common and usually minor form of mental disorder experienced in some form or other by most people. It may be caused by some *anxiety* or experience (trauma), or by unre-

Sex Problems and Sexuality

solved conflicts. Symptoms of neurosis may resemble fatigue, nervousness, *depression*, fear, *obsession* or *hysteria*.

Obsession. A common form of *neurosis* characterized by a recurring idea that compels the individual to do something to relieve an exaggerated sense of anxiety. It is most likely to occur in a minor form. Severe forms of obsession may cause great inconvenience, and may develop to the point where they dominate the waking hours of the patient's life.

Paranoia. A severe mental disorder in which delusions of persecution affect a person's way of life and reactions to outside situations. The characteristics of a paranoic include suspicion, self-consciousness, and logical explanations of the delusions, which support an increasing web of dislikes and fears. Paranoia may be dangerous because the patient believes that the persecution is real, and so may act violently as a result of this delusion.

TREATMENT. Psychiatric therapy is necessary to rehabilitate mild cases. Severe cases require permanent care.

Psychosis. An abnormal mental state produced by *alcoholism, schizophrenia,* addictive drugs or an underlying illness. Psychosis is indicated by major disorders of personality, often associated with delusions, hallucinations and abnormal behaviour.

TREATMENT. Hospitalization is usually required.

Schizophrenia. A mental disorder affecting emotion and thought and, ultimately, behaviour. The causes of the disorder are not known, but it has been attributed to various influences, including hereditary factors, chemical imbalance in the brain, upbringing, emotional stress, and *drug abuse*.

TREATMENT. Initially, specialized psychiatric care is required to give the patient confidence in a shared, rather than an isolated, sense of reality. If this is not successful the patient may need compulsory hospital treatment and the use of anti-psychotic and tranquillizing drugs. Continued psychiatric care is usually required to prevent relapse.

Sex Problems and Sexuality

Abnormal development. If a child's normal *sexuality* is frustrated, feelings of guilt and inhibition occur. These tend to prevent normal adult sexual development and leave the individual with underlying sexual desires that remain frustrated and in need of fulfilment. Various aspects of abnormal sexual development are discussed below.

Exhibitionism in young children is a form of infantile sexuality in which the child exhibits its genitals in order to attract a parent. In an adult male, it is an expression of his fear and dislike of women. A similar sexual gratification is sought by the voyeur, who observes a person of the opposite sex undressing, either in commercial strip-tease shows or through the window of a private house.

Fetishism originally described the worship of an object imbued with supernatural power. It is now used more commonly to refer to the sexual attraction to objects associated with sex. Fetishism, in certain cases, may be the only form in which sexual satisfaction can be attained, or it may simply be an aid to sexual activity.

Narcissism is a form of excessive self-love. It is a stage in the sexual development of all children which usually passes

Sex Problems and Sexuality

as the child progresses to more satisfying social relationships. If the stage persists, however, it may prevent the development of satisfactory adult relationships.

Paedophilia is a sexual love for children. Avoidance of the responsibilities of adult relationships may lead to misinterpretation of a simple, loving relationship with a child as an ideal sexual relationship. The child may respond with a similar love and this can cause the child to suffer emotional problems when the relationship is broken. In its extreme form, in which the child is molested sexually, it is illegal.

All serious problems due to failure of normal sexual development need skilled psychiatric care. Psychoanalysis may be needed to find the point at which normal development was frustrated, before any real help can be given.

Physical problems. The inability to take part in sexual activities because of a physical difficulty. The problem may be one of ignorance or anxiety about the physical techniques of sexual intercourse, in which case simple explanations given by a doctor are all that are required. If intercourse is painful it may be due to a disorder of the vagina, or to some other female problem, or it may be caused by an inflammation of the end of the penis. In either case, consult a doctor. The problem may also be one of physical disability. Paralysis, a nerve disorder such as sciatica, arthritis, or illnesses such as diabetes may lead to sexual problems, any of which should be discussed with a doctor.

Psychological problems. Almost all aspects of sexuality are affected by a person's mentality, adolescent experience and present state of mind. Depression produces a lack of sexual drive and reduces the frequency of intercourse. This requires sympathy and understanding from the healthy partner, and treatment of the cause of depression. Sexual frustration may occur if there is no normal sexual relief, and can lead to depression, anxiety and irritability. In institutions containing people of only one sex, frustration may lead to masturbation and homosexuality and may occasionally lead to violent sexual attacks. In most circumstances, a mild form of sexual inhibition is normal, so that sexuality does not disturb everyday social contact. Excessive sexuality, known in women as nymphomania and in men as satyriasis, may occur as a result of failure to establish a lasting satisfactory relationship. It may also be a symptom of mania, psychotic mental illness or occasionally excessive hormonal activity.

Vaginismus is a painful tightening of a woman's pelvic muscles around the vagina that prevents sexual intercourse. This usually has a psychological basis such as fear about sexual intercourse. Frigidity, a complete lack of sexual interest, may be associated with fear of pregnancy, venereal disease or pain, or with the belief that sexual intercourse is immoral. Failure of orgasm in women may be a mild form of frigidity but it may also indicate fatigue, illness or another minor disorder in a normally happy relationship.

Erection problems (impotence) may occur in a man for psychological reasons. Premature ejaculation of sperm frequently occurs in men when they are sexually inexperienced, anxious or if they feel guilty about sex.

Homosexuality is sexual attraction for someone of the same sex. In women it is known as lesbianism. It is a normal stage in the development of sexuality and many people maintain happy and contented homosexual relationships without any need for heterosexual intercourse. Some people are bisexual, having sexual relationships with both sexes. Variations in sexual behaviour become psychological problems only where they cause anxiety or guilt. Oral sex, anal sex and sex involving the use of slight pain (sadism or masochism) are common. In extreme forms such variations are abnormal and can be dangerous.

Incest is an illegal sexual relationship with a close relative, such as father with daughter, mother with son, or brother with sister. It is particularly likely to occur in social circumstances in which members of a family are forced into unusually close contact with each other.

Sexuality. The complicated association of natural instincts leading to the desire for sexual reproduction. Sexuality is specifically used to describe the psychological and physical responses of one person in sexual relation to another. This feeling of attraction and compatibility varies greatly between people and is modified by different circumstances. A child learns how to attract and respond to parents and friends before puberty. After puberty these subtle patterns are used with strangers and help to establish new friendships, some of which may be physically sexual, until a permanent relationship is formed that may lead to marriage.

The self-stimulation of sexual areas to produce an orgasm (masturbation) is a common and normal method of obtaining relief from the feeling of physical sexual tension when sexual intercourse is not possible. It starts during infancy and becomes more frequent at puberty. It can produce feelings of guilt if the child is reprimanded and can make the child feel that sexuality is, in some way, unhealthy or bad. This may distort normal sexual development in a child and lead to frigidity or impotence in an adult.

Skin Problems

Abscess (boil, carbuncle, furuncle). A tissue infection in which pus forms. A boil or furuncle is an infection of a sweat gland or hair follicle, and a carbuncle is a large abscess, or boil, with several openings.

TREATMENT. A small boil can be treated with local heat, from a warm compress or a heated spoon, at regular intervals until the boil bursts, when a dry dressing should be applied. A large boil or abscess should be covered with a dry dressing and seen by a doctor as soon as possible because it may require treatment with antibiotics.

Acne. A chronic skin condition of the face and shoulders. It is most common in adolescence, and is probably caused by a combination of factors, including the type of skin and hormonal stimulus of puberty. Sweat glands are more easily blocked if the skin is greasy, forming blackheads (comedos), the typical spots of acne. Bacteria may infect the blocked gland so that it becomes inflamed. Occasionally acne can lead to recurrent *abscess* formation and leave *scars*.

TREATMENT. A healthy diet, avoiding sweets and rich or spicy foods, and taking regular exercise in the open air prevent serious acne. Do not squeeze the spots, as this spreads any infection. Wash the hair regularly, two or three times a

Skin Problems

week. Wash the face, fingernails and hands several times a day. If these simple measures fail, consult a doctor.

Bedsore. Ulceration of the skin on the buttocks, heels, elbows or shoulders in a bedridden patient. It is caused by lying in one position for too long. This restricts the blood supply to the affected area, which turns blue-black and ulcerates.

TREATMENT. Bedsores are prevented by regular movement, by rubbing the area with surgical spirit and powder, by keeping the skin dry, and by improving general health, with additional vitamins if necessary. Once a bedsore has formed there must be no further pressure on it and the area should be cleaned with an antiseptic solution.

Birthmark. A blemish present at birth. Moles are common and seldom need treatment but birthmarks on the legs and those that undergo sudden change in size or colour should be seen by a doctor. They can be removed by minor surgery.

Body odour (bromhidrosis). Odour caused by the decomposition of dead skin cells and sweat by skin bacteria. It can be aggravated by anxiety, which increases sweating, or by a spiced diet.

TREATMENT. Daily bathing and change of underclothes are important. The use of antiperspirant and deodorant preparations may also help.

Chloasma. A patchy brown pigmentation of the forehead and cheeks. It sometimes occurs during pregnancy, and may also result from taking the contraceptive pill or from disorders of the adrenal gland. In most cases it improves spontaneously. If it does not, or if it causes embarrassment, consult a doctor.

Cyst, sebaceous. Blockage of a grease gland may be followed by cyst formation if the gland continues to secrete. This happens more commonly in some people than in others. Symptoms include painless swelling, just under the skin, most commonly on the scalp, at the back of the neck and on the shoulders. The size increases slowly over several years and occasionally may discharge a soft cheese-like material before continuing to swell.

TREATMENT. If it is unsightly or in a place where it rubs against clothing, surgical removal (under local anaesthetic) may be required.

Dermatitis. Inflammation of the skin. It may have a variety of causes such as an allergy, anxiety, *eczema,* or contact with irritating poisons or other chemicals, including certain cosmetics and detergents. Symptoms include redness, itching and sometimes other lesions such as blisters.

TREATMENT. Consult a doctor to determine the cause. Skin lotions may remove the inflammation.

Eczema. An itching skin eruption for which there is no external cause. It is related to allergic conditions such as hay fever, nettle rash and asthma. It may affect babies from about four months. Typically, a red, scaling rash appears on the scalp, spreads to the cheeks and to the limbs, particularly in front of the elbows and behind the knees. An intense itching causes scratching and insomnia. The condition varies greatly from time to time and may be aggravated by heat, cold and certain foods. Measles and chickenpox tend to be more severe than usual and affected children must not be vaccinated against smallpox because the reaction may be fatal. Eczema may occur in adults, particularly if the person is under stress.

TREATMENT. During an attack, antihistamine drugs and corticosteroid creams may be used, following a doctor's advice. Cotton clothing and gloves worn at night to prevent scratching are advisable for young children. A normal diet is recommended unless an allergy to some food is suspected.

Impetigo. A contagious infection occurring around the mouth and nose. It affects children in particular. Symptoms include blisters that form crusts and spread across the face, hands or knees. The infection is usually more severe in people who suffer from *eczema*.

TREATMENT. Consult a doctor for an appropriate antibiotic ointment. Cleanliness of body, hands and nails is necessary to prevent a recurrence of the disease.

Lice (nits, crabs). Small parasites that infest the skin of mammals and birds. They bite to suck blood from the host and cause itching and scratching. The eggs are often laid in the host's hair. Three types affect humans. Head lice (nits) are most often encountered in children. They are not an indication of lack of cleanliness so much as of shared clothes and towels, usually at school. Body lice are more commonly associated with a lack of hygiene. These are the parasites which are usually responsible for the spread of typhus, plague, and other infectious illnesses. The third type of louse is the pubic or crab louse which inhabits the hairs of the pubic region and is transmitted by sexual contact. The names of these parasites indicate the region in which they are usually found, but each type may also be encountered elsewhere.

TREATMENT. Insecticide powder, anti-louse shampoos and lotions and careful removal of eggs help to eradicate the parasites. If lice remain, consult a doctor.

Moniliasis (candidiasis). A fungus infection that develops in warm, moist areas of the body. It is responsible for thrush infections of the vagina or mouth, but may also affect the skin, particularly in the groin, under the breasts and around the fingernails.

TREATMENT. Keep the affected area as dry as possible. Antifungal ointments, powders and tablets are available, following a doctor's advice.

Nettle rash (urticaria). A transient eruption of pale, itching swellings. It may be caused by jellyfish or nettle stings, insect bites, a mild allergy to certain foods or drugs, or it may be a reaction to emotions such as anxiety and depression.

TREATMENT. A cold compress, a soothing lotion, and antihistamine drugs, often relieve the symptoms.

Psoriasis. A skin disease, characterized by patches of mildly irritated, red, scaling skin. The cause of psoriasis is not known. The symptoms may not appear until adulthood, and they may vary greatly in severity, sometimes disappearing for long periods of time. They are likely to be aggravated by emotional stress.

TREATMENT. Various skin preparations may help to reduce scaling. Sunlight is beneficial and the use of various strong, cell-killing (cytotoxic) drugs may help severe cases.

Rash. A pink or red, often itching, inflammation of the skin. It is usually a sign of an allergic reaction, in which case it is of short duration. It may also be a symptom of certain infectious illnesses, such as measles and chickenpox, or of a skin infection, and it may be associated with anxiety.

Skin Problems

TREATMENT. It is important to treat the allergy or disease that causes the rash. Cooling the inflamed area and applying a soothing lotion may give temporary relief.

Scabies. A contagious skin infection transmitted by mites. It is spread by close body contact and is easily passed from one member of a family to another. The mite burrows into the skin, usually in the hand or wrist, pubic area, elbows or buttocks. After about a month a red rash appears in the infected area as an allergic reaction. People who are subsequently reinfected develop the rash within a few hours because the allergy is already present.

TREATMENT. After a bath, dry carefully and paint the whole body, from neck downwards, with an anti-scabies preparation. Repeat on the two following days. Change bed linen and clothing and wash the used fabrics with great care.

Scars. Inelastic tissue formed as part of the normal healing process of cut or damaged skin. Keloid scars are thicker than normal because too much fibrous tissue has been produced. These occur after burns, in particular, and in some people who are particularly susceptible. Contraction of large scars may prevent full movement of a joint and such scars often distort the tissues of the face. An irregular, thick, contracted scar may be made less unsightly by plastic surgery.

Tinea (ringworm). A fungus infection of the skin. It is usually contracted in communal wash-places such as school and sports club shower-rooms and swimming pools, from contaminated damp towels and wet floors. Occasionally animal ringworm is caught from close contact with sheep, cattle, dogs or cats. Tinea may infect the creases between the toes (athlete's foot), the groin, the armpits, the nails and, occasionally, the scalp. Animal ringworm tends to cause large rings, with slightly raised edges, anywhere on the skin. Normally ringworm is a mildly irritating red patch which becomes sore when moist.

TREATMENT. Antifungal creams and powders usually cure athlete's foot but other areas may need more specific medical attention. Infection of the nails requires prolonged therapy with antifungal drugs.

Verrucas and warts. Small tumours of the skin caused by a virus infection. Warts and verrucas are commonest in children aged between eight and 12 and occur most commonly as small growths on the hands but also on the face and the soles of the feet. The term verruca is commonly used for a wart on the sole of the foot (plantar wart), where pressure on it is painful. Most warts disappear spontaneously within a year without treatment.

TREATMENT. Consult a doctor. If necessary warts can be removed by cutting them out, by burning them with acid, or by freezing them with carbon dioxide snow.

Systemic and General Problems

Allergy. A state of unusual physical sensitivity to certain substances. Allergies can occur only when the body has encountered the allergenic substance before. An extremely severe allergic reaction is known as *anaphylaxis*.

TREATMENT. Symptoms may be controlled by antihistamines, by cromoglycate preparations, and sometimes by corticosteroid drugs.

Systemic and General Problems

Anaphylaxis. A very severe allergic reaction, usually to a drug
[H] or to an insect sting. The patient may feel faint, vomit and be
incontinent, or collapse and become unconscious. Breathing
may be difficult (wheezing). Extreme pallor is likely because
of reduced blood pressure due to shock.

TREATMENT. A doctor or an ambulance must be called at
once. An inhalation from the type of aerosol used by asthma-
tics can help and the doctor may give an injection of adrenalin
and antihistamine.

Cancer. A condition in which the normal restrictions on cell
growth in a particular area of the body are diminished or lost.
Without these restrictions, cells grow to form a *tumour*. Local
growth continues and cells may spread to other areas of the
body through the lymphatic system and the blood. Tumours
which grow at a distance from the original growth in this way
are called metastatic tumours.

In many cases the exact cause of cancer is not known. Environmental causes, such as smoking, working in some chemical industries, and excessive sunlight (which may produce
skin cancer and rodent ulcers), are common. It is likely that
some chemical substances in foods induce cancer and certain
forms of cooking, such as frying in fat, may also encourage
cancer formation. Virus infections produce cancer in animals
and may cause some kinds of leukaemia in man. Some diseases, such as ulcerative colitis and cirrhosis, may sometimes
produce cancer in the area affected.

Cancer, in its early stages, is curable. The problem is to
discover it before it has spread. This depends on the patient
reporting to a doctor any change in the normal working of the
body. The skin is easy to watch, and any mole or wart that
changes colour or size must be shown to a doctor. A persistent
cough, particularly in a smoker, needs a thorough assessment. The appearance of blood in the urine, a change in bowel
habit and, in women, unusual vaginal bleeding around the
time of the menopause may all be suspicious symptoms. A
woman should examine her breasts once a month, after her
period, with the flat of the hand to feel for breast lumps.

Later symptoms of cancer include loss of weight, general
malaise and pain. These usually occur after the minor
symptoms have been ignored but occasionally the cancer is so
hidden that it does not cause any early symptoms and this is
the reason why cancer diagnosis may be so difficult. Diagnosis of cancer requires the full facilities of a hospital. X-
rays, blood tests and the removal of suspicious parts of a
tumour for microscopic analysis may all be required before
the diagnosis is confirmed and treatment is started.

TREATMENT. Cancer can be treated in various ways and often
a combination of these must be used. Treatment may include
an operation to remove the growth, X-ray treatment
(radiotherapy) to destroy the tumour cells, and cancer-
killing drugs (chemotherapy) given by mouth or by injection.
There are many kinds of cancer and so no single treatment
can be used with success in all cases. Early diagnosis and
treatment are most important, but the type of tumour, its
location and the likelihood of rapid spread are also significant. Careful follow-up study ensures that any recurrence
is found quickly so that further treatment can be given before
damage is done. The treatment of cancer is improving each

Systemic and General Problems

year. Anxiety should not prevent anyone seeking help, because what is feared as cancer is often something much less serious. Only a thorough examination will determine whether cancer is present or not and if it is dangerous. The sooner a diagnosis is made, the sooner treatment can begin.

Diabetes. A general name for related diseases characterized by excessive urination. Diabetes insipidus is a rare disorder due to a lack of pituitary antidiuretic hormone or to a kidney abnormality. It usually responds to treatment with antidiuretic hormone replacement. Diabetes mellitus (sugar diabetes) may develop suddenly as a result of an acute infection of the pancreas or gradually, resulting from an inherited tendency, from obesity, from excessive alcohol or from increasing age. There is a failure to control sugar in the body due to a lack of insulin, which is normally produced by the pancreas. Symptoms include thirst, excessive urination, lethargy and, rarely, coma. Diagnosis is made by testing for sugar in the urine and for an excessive level in the blood.

TREATMENT. Mild cases may be treated by lowering sugar in the diet and reducing weight. If this fails, tablets may be taken to stimulate insulin production. Insulin injections are given only if diet and tablets do not succeed or if the onset of the disease is sudden and severe. The dosage is adjusted to the individual's requirements and is usually given once or twice a day. Excessive doses of insulin may reduce the blood's sugar level too far, and cause weakness, sweating, trembling, confusion and sometimes loss of consciousness (hypoglycaemic coma). This is rapidly improved by eating sugar or by an injection of glucose given by a doctor.

All diabetics, on drugs or insulin, should carry a card stating their name, the required dosage of insulin and what to do if they are found unconscious.

Fever. The normal human body temperature varies with the time of day, within a range from 96°F (35.5°C) to 98.6°F (37°C) or even a little higher. The normal mouth temperature (98.6°F, 37°C) is often exceeded following physical activity, particularly in hot weather. Babies and children have a greater range of normal temperature. The temperature in the rectum is usually about 1°F (0.5°C) higher than in the mouth.

A fever is a temperature of 100°F (37.7°C) or higher that continues for more than four hours. Babies and children tend to have higher fevers than do adults. Fever may be caused by almost any general infection of the body, and by some physical conditions. The sudden onset of a high temperature (104°F, 40°C) may be accompanied by a rigor and followed by excessive sweating which is the chief means by which the body can lose heat. High fevers may be accompanied by confusion or delirium. In infants they can cause convulsions. Slight fevers are usually recognized before the temperature is measured by a sense of chill and general *malaise*.

TREATMENT. If the patient has a high temperature (104°F, 40°C) and is confused, vomiting or complaining of a severe headache, a doctor should be consulted at once. In other cases it is often best to use simple treatments and measure the temperature again in two or three hours. A fever is only one of the signs of illness and other symptoms should be taken into account. In all cases a doctor should be consulted if a fever persists. Simple treatments for a fever that can be

118

Systemic and General Problems

carried out at home include soluble aspirin, bed rest, generous consumption of fluids, light diet and cool sponging if the temperature rises above 103°F (39.4°C).

Malaise (listlessness, fatigue). Vague symptoms associated with most illnesses, particularly if the onset of an illness or disease is gradual. Listlessness is a characteristic symptom of recovery from an illness or an operation, but in some cases is associated with depression.

TREATMENT. Continued listlessness, without obvious cause, requires medical examination. If there is a suspected cause, consult a doctor for advice about the best means of treating it.

Night sweats. These are common in healthy children who have been active all day and whose body temperature drops suddenly when asleep. A night sweat is normal even if it is so severe that the child's night-clothes are soaked. Night sweats may also occur in adults who use too many bedclothes or keep an electric blanket on at night. They may also occur in any illness that is associated with *fever*. If they occur irregularly over a long period, consult a doctor.

Rheumatic fever. An allergic reaction, related to acute nephritis and scarlet fever, that affects the heart and joints of children. It is caused by a streptococcal infection. Symptoms include a sore throat followed about two weeks later by fever, with intermittent painful swelling of the joints. Sometimes there is a blotchy rash. All layers of the heart, including the valves, are likely to be involved. The disease lasts many weeks, and the damage to the heart may be permanent.

TREATMENT. Bed rest with large doses of aspirin and nursing care of the joints are required for the duration of the illness. Antibiotics may be required for several years. The patient needs thorough medical assessment.

Thyroid problems. The thyroid gland lies in front of the windpipe (trachea) in the neck. Hormones from the thyroid, particularly thyroxine, control the speed of activity (metabolism) of the cells of the body.

Over-production of thyroxine is known as hyperthyroidism. Symptoms include palpitations, sweating, large appetite but loss of weight, sometimes diarrhoea and menstrual disorders, protruding eyes, and trembling hands. A lack of thyroxine (hypothyroidism or myxoedema) sometimes occurs after treatment for hyperthyroidism, but it is also associated with increasing age and thyroid failure. Babies born with too little thyroxine may suffer from cretinism, causing mental retardation. Symptoms of hypothyroidism include lethargy, mental slowing, complaints of cold, hair falling out and coarsening of the skin.

TREATMENT. For hyperthyroidism, younger patients are given pills to reduce thyroid activity. This may be followed by an operation to remove part of the thyroid gland. Older patients are usually treated with radioactive iodine. This is safe but it may eventually lead to hypothroidism. For hypothyroidism, consult a doctor, who will usually give thyroxine tablets.

Tumour. A lump or swelling in the body tissues. It may be due to an infection such as a boil, to local damage such as a bruise or to an abnormal growth of body tissue. This abnormal growth may be due to cancer or it may be a benign growth such as a lipoma or a fibrous tissue swelling (fibroma).

Systemic and General Problems

TREATMENT. There are many types of tumour, and so each must be diagnosed carefully for the appropriate treatment. If you find an abnormal swelling you should consult a doctor. Tumours in the breast may be detected by monthly examination with the flat of the hand. See *Breast Problems: Breast examination*.

Vitamins. Essential substances, small amounts of which are required in the diet for the normal working of the body. They are classified in two main groups, those that dissolve in fat and those that dissolve in water.

Vitamin A. A fat-soluble vitamin found in liver, cod liver oil, butter and eggs. It is necessary for vision in poor light and for a healthy skin. Deficiency leads to night blindness and dry skin. An excess may cause liver damage, drowsiness and headache.

Vitamin B_1 (thiamin). A water-soluble vitamin found in milk, eggs, wholemeal bread and fruit. It is necessary for the metabolism of carbohydrates. Deficiency leads to beri-beri, either wet with heart failure or dry with polyneuritis.

Vitamin B_2 (riboflavin). A water-soluble vitamin found in milk, liver, yeast, kidney and eggs, necessary for releasing energy from food. Deficiency, which is rare, causes soreness at the corners of the mouth.

Nicotinic acid (niacin). A water-soluble vitamin of the B group, found in bread, milk, vegetables and meat. It is important for preventing the skin condition pellagra.

Vitamin B_6 (pyridoxin). A water-soluble vitamin found in most foods, particularly meat, eggs, fish and flour. It is necessary for the formation of body protein. Symptoms of deficiency are rare, but may include anaemia.

Vitamin B_{12}. A water-soluble vitamin found in liver, eggs and cheese, important for normal blood production and healthy nerve tissue. Deficiency leads to pernicious anaemia and polyneuritis.

Folic acid. A water-soluble vitamin found in liver, kidney and leaf vegetables, required for normal blood production. Deficiency leads to anaemia.

Pantothenic acid and biotin. Water-soluble vitamins found in most foods, used in the formation of body fats. Deficiency does not occur.

Vitamin C (ascorbic acid). A water-soluble vitamin found in green vegetables, fruit and potatoes. It is necessary to keep body tissues adherent to each other. Deficiency leads to scurvy, in which the tissues tend to disintegrate.

Vitamin D. A fat-soluble vitamin found in cod liver oil, fatty fish, eggs, milk and butter. It is needed to maintain the calcium level in blood and bone. Deficiency leads to rickets and osteomalacia, caused by softening of the bone. An excess causes too much calcium to be absorbed and this can damage kidney tissue, particularly of children, and occasionally other parts of the body such as the tendons.

Vitamin E. A fat-soluble vitamin found in most foods, particularly vegetable oils, eggs and flour. Its value is uncertain.

Vitamin K. A fat-soluble vitamin found in leaf vegetables, pulses and cereals. It is synthesized in the intestine, and is required for the normal clotting mechanisms of the blood. Deficiency rarely occurs except with severe liver disease or following the use of certain drugs.

Urogenital Problems

Contraception. Contraception prevents a pregnancy from occurring. Many different methods and devices are used but not all of these are equally effective.

There are several forms of contraception for use by men. The sheath (condom) is an efficient form of contraception if properly used, preferably with spermicidal vaginal creams, foams or gels. Coitus interruptus (withdrawal before ejaculation) is not safe as sperm may have been produced during the earlier stages of intercourse. Vasectomy or male sterilization is a completely effective form of contraception. It is a small operation, usually done under local anaesthetic, in which the spermatic cord is cut and the ends tied. Vasectomy does not interfere with sex drive or ability and does not cause any physical side-effects but the operation is difficult to reverse.

There are more methods and devices for women than there are for men. The diaphragm or Dutch cap is a special rubber cap designed to be placed over the entrance (cervix) to the womb to prevent sperm from entering. It does not harm the woman and cannot be felt by the man. If a diaphragm is properly used, with spermicidal creams, it is an effective form of contraception. Proper use of the diaphragm has to be learnt and it must be fitted some time before intercourse and left in place for at least eight hours afterwards.

An intra-uterine contraceptive device (IUCD or IUD) is a metal (copper or platinum) or plastic coil, ring or other shape that prevents the fertilized egg from settling in the lining of the womb. It is an extremely safe form of contraception, better than the diaphragm, but it may cause painful, heavy menstruation (sometimes leading to anaemia) or it may introduce infection.

The contraceptive pill is regarded as the most effective form of contraception. It is usually made from the synthetic equivalents of two hormones, oestrogen and progesterone, or from the progesterone-like hormone by itself. It is a pill that is taken daily for three weeks of a four-week cycle. Menstruation usually occurs in the fourth week. Its main hazard is that it may cause thrombosis and this danger is greatly increased in those who have a history of previous thrombosis, diabetes, high blood pressure, liver disease, varicose veins, cancer of the breast or epilepsy, and in those over the age of 35. Failure to take the pill on one night should be rectified by taking two pills the following night. Missing more than one night means that protection is no longer effective and the packet should be thrown away and a new packet started after seven days without the pill. In such cases protection is not certain for the first 14 days of the new cycle. It is common for there to be no menstruation for six to eight weeks after stopping the pill and it is possible to become pregnant during this time if no other precautions are taken. A doctor should be consulted if menstruation does not start.

The "safe period" is a method of calculating the probable time of ovulation and avoiding intercourse at this time. It is not really safe because it only reduces the chances of pregnancy and does nothing positive to prevent it. Contraceptive foams, creams and gels are inserted into the vagina to kill the sperm. These are not safe by themselves

Urogenital Problems

although they may be used effectively with a diaphragm or sheath.

Salpingectomy or sterilization of a woman is an effective means of contraception, but one that is difficult to reverse. The Fallopian tubes are cut and tied or clipped, either at an abdominal operation or by a technique using a special instrument (laparoscope) which can examine the abdominal contents through a small incision. See also *Gynaecological Problems: Contraceptive problems*.

Cystitis. An inflammation of the bladder. The infection may spread down the ureter from a kidney infection or up the urethra from an infection such as vaginitis or diarrhoea. Cystitis is much more common in women than in men because the female urethra is shorter. Symptoms include burning discomfort and frequent urination, sometimes with blood in the urine, and fever in severe cases. Some attacks of recurrent cystitis are caused by sexual intercourse, because the massaging effect forces an infection into the bladder. This may be prevented by the woman emptying her bladder after intercourse and by careful washing. Recurring attacks of cystitis must be discussed with a doctor.

TREATMENT. Drink large amounts of fluid to dilute the urine. In more serious cases antibiotic, antispasm and painkilling drugs may be prescribed. Local infections, such as vaginitis or skin problems, should also be treated.

Foreskin, sore (balanitis). This is common in babies and is associated with nappy rash. In adults it may occur in the uncircumcised due to poor hygiene or friction against wet clothing.

TREATMENT. Consult a doctor for the appropriate antiseptic or antibiotic treatment. Circumcision may be required if there is recurrent infection.

Incontinence. The inability to hold urine because of failure to control the sphincter muscle that closes the opening from the bladder into the urethra. It is a problem of the elderly but may also affect men who suffer from *prostate problems* and women in whom the bladder is compressed, either during pregnancy, or by a prolapse of the womb. Incontinence usually occurs if the bladder is compressed when laughing or coughing. It may also occur during sleep.

TREATMENT. Consult a doctor. Treatment will depend on the cause but if incontinence occurs as a result of prostate or gynaecological problems an operation may be required.

Kidney disorders. The body's blood supply is filtered by the two kidneys to maintain the correct balance of water and salts. Waste substances, such as urea and uric acid, are excreted with the excess of salt and water. Symptoms of kidney disease include back pain, urination problems, blood or pus in the urine, and fever. Kidney disease may be detected by examination of the blood and urine and by X-rays following the injection of a dye into the circulation. This test, an intravenous pyelogram, depends on the dye being detected by the X-rays as it is excreted through the kidneys.

Congenital abnormalities of the kidneys, such as cysts, double kidneys and double ureters, may all occur and these make infection or stone formation more likely.

TREATMENT. In all cases a doctor must be consulted, and hospitalization for assessment of the disorder is usually required. See also *Nephritis* and *Pyelonephritis*.

Urogenital Problems

Moniliasis (candidiasis, thrush). A fungal infection that is particularly likely to affect the vagina, although it can develop in other parts of the body as well. It causes itching and vaginal discharge. The fungus can also affect the male who carries the infection even though he may feel no symptoms.

TREATMENT. Consult a doctor. Antifungal creams and ointments may be prescribed. If a woman is treated for the infection her sexual partner should also receive treatment because the fungus may remain alive in the penis and reinfect the woman when her treatment has stopped.

Nephritis. An inflammation of the kidney. Symptoms include back pain, swollen eyelids and ankles, rapid pulse, fever, vomiting and dark, blood-stained urine.

TREATMENT. A doctor must be consulted and hospitalization is often required. Absolute bed rest is essential, with a diet that is low in protein and salt. Antibiotics may be given to prevent the infection spreading to other parts of the body.

Prostate problems. The prostate gland is found in men underneath the bladder. As the urethra passes through the gland from the bladder to the penis, it is joined by the two spermatic cords from the testes.

Prostatic enlargement occurs as men get older, and is fairly common over the age of 60. The enlargement distorts the bladder and the urethra. Symptoms of prostatic enlargement include frequent or difficult urination, together with hesitant starting and dribbling after finishing. Sometimes an urgent need to urinate is followed by an inability to do so. Slight *incontinence*, sometimes complete retention of urine, and occasionally blood in the urine may also occur. An infection of the prostate (prostatitis) may occur at any age and may be a complication of veneral diseases such as gonorrhoea. The symptoms resemble those of prostatic enlargement.

TREATMENT. Consult a doctor because increasingly severe symptoms indicate that an operation is required. This is usually performed through the penis but may sometimes be performed through the abdomen. If cancer is found, drug treatment is often effective. Infections of the prostate are usually treated with antibiotics.

Pyelonephritis. Inflammation of the pelvis of the kidney. It may be caused by pregnancy, *cystitis*, tuberculosis, a congenital abnormality or an obstruction to the urine flow. Symptoms include fever, chill, frequent and painful urination, backache and vomiting.

TREATMENT. Antibiotic therapy, pain-killing drugs and bed rest are necessary for recovery. If the infection is not completely cleared it may cause chronic pyelitis and gradual kidney damage leading to kidney failure.

Stone in kidney. Stones may be formed from excess salts and uric acid. They are usually caused by a lack of fluid in hot climates, gout, infection, or congenital abnormalities. There are often no symptoms unless the stone moves and causes an obstruction. In such cases colic, severe backache, spasmodic pain in the groin, vomiting, sweating, and frequent urination with evidence of blood in the urine may occur.

TREATMENT. Call a doctor as soon as symptoms develop. Strong pain-killing and antispasm drugs may be required. An intravenous pyelogram, described under *Kidney disorders,* shows the position of the stone. It may be possible to

Urogenital Problems

remove the stone through the bladder but if this fails, an abdominal operation may be necessary.

Urination, frequent. This may be a symptom of diabetes, but it may also occur in pregnancy, because of pressure on the bladder by the growing fetus, and in an older woman whose bladder and the ligaments supporting it have been damaged by pregnancy. Frequent urination may also be a symptom of anxiety or of *cystitis*. If the condition persists for more than two days, with no obvious cause, consult a doctor.

Urine, blood in (haematuria). This may be a symptom of *cystitis* or *prostate problems*, if it is associated with pain on urination, or it may be a symptom of *nephritis* or *pyelonephritis* if there is also back pain or fever. Stones or growths in the bladder or kidney may cause painless haematuria.

TREATMENT. Consult a doctor as soon as possible, and take a sample of urine for examination.

Urine, discoloration of. The urine is naturally darker in the morning, during a fever and if one is dehydrated. It is very dark in some illnesses, such as jaundice, and may also be darkened by some drugs. Sometimes a milky discoloration occurs due to the crystallization of salts in concentrated urine, but this is not serious. The smell of urine varies with concentration and diet, but a strong fishy smell is often associated with *cystitis* and urinary infections.

TREATMENT. If the urine appears unusually dark or cloudy, increase the amount of fluids drunk. If the discoloration or strange smell persists, consult a doctor for advice, taking a sample of the urine for examination.

Urine, retention of. The inability to urinate, despite feeling the need to do so, may indicate *prostate problems*, or *cystitis* if the retention is associated with pain. It may also be a sign of a neurological problem such as a stroke and it is common after an operation, particularly a gynaecological one, in which local bruising causes this temporary reaction.

TREATMENT. A hot bath, or the sound of running water may help urination to occur. Pain-killing drugs such as aspirin may be useful. If these measures fail, consult a doctor. Hospital admission may be required for a tube (catheter) to be passed into the bladder to drain the urine.

Venereal Diseases

Chancre. An ulcer, the first sign of syphilis, that appears about three weeks after catching the disease. It is a slightly raised area with a depressed centre, but it is not tender. It occurs on the penis, vulva, internally on the cervix, or occasionally on the mouth. It will disappear in three to four weeks, leaving only a small scar. Great care must be taken during the chancre stage of syphilis because it is then highly contagious, and the chancre itself contains the organisms of this disease.

TREATMENT. Cover with a dry dressing and consult a doctor urgently.

Chancroid (soft sore). A highly infectious non-syphilitic ulcer, common in tropical countries. A chancroid ulcer is tender and yellow. Local lymph glands become inflamed, full of pus and may discharge. The disease may affect the penis, urethra, vulva and anus, and usually spreads rapidly.

TREATMENT. Consult a doctor immediately. This disease usually responds well to treatment with antibiotics.

Venereal Diseases

Gonorrhoea. A contagious sexually transmitted bacterial infection of the genital mucous membranes of either sex. Inflammation appears within a week of contracting the disease. Gonorrhoea may also affect other parts of the body such as the conjunctiva and oral mucosa, rectum or joints. In the male, gonorrhoea may cause pain on urination and be detected by a milky discharge from the *penis.* Although the disease may not cause symptoms in the female, vaginal discharge and tenderness are often present.

TREATMENT. Avoid further sexual intercourse and consult a doctor. Penicillin is the most effective treatment but occasionally the infecting bacteria is resistant and other antibiotics must be used.

Granuloma inguinale. A bacterial infection that is most common in tropical countries. The sign of infection is a small nodule in the genital area which slowly begins to ulcerate.

TREATMENT. Consult a doctor. Treatment with antibiotics is usually effective.

Herpes genitalis. A virus, causing an infection like a cold sore in the genital region. It is usually but not always transmitted through sexual intercourse. Symptoms include painful blisters in the genital region which become inflamed.

TREATMENT. After seven to ten days the sores will begin to disappear. Cold compresses and pain-killing drugs may help. A doctor must be consulted.

Non-specific urethritis (NSU). Inflammation of the urethra not due to any specific infection. NSU is transmitted through sexual intercourse but is caused by non-gonorrhoeal organisms. Symptoms resemble those of gonorrhoea. In men they include painful urination and discharge from the *penis.* In women symptoms include a red and swollen vulva and a discharge of pus from the vagina and the urethra.

TREATMENT. Consult a doctor. The discharge must be examined so that the cause of infection can be identified. Treatment with antibiotics may be required.

Penis, discharge from. This is always a sign of infection. It may be caused by any venereal disease, but most commonly it is due to *gonorrhoea.*

TREATMENT. Both patient and sexual partner must consult a doctor and abstain from sexual intercourse until cured.

Syphilis. The most serious of venereal diseases, syphilis is caused by the organism Treponema pallidum, usually transmitted through sexual intercourse. The chief symptom of the primary stage is *chancre* which appears within three weeks of contracting the disease. The second stage, which occurs six or eight weeks later, is indicated by a mild fever, a rash over the body, swollen lymph glands, sore throat and headache. The third stage may not occur for 10 to 15 years. Swellings in any tissue may develop and interfere with the normal workings of the body. The final stage involves the nervous system and causes the condition known as general paralysis of the insane, symptoms of which include loss of sensation in the legs, a staggering gait and ulceration of the skin.

TREATMENT. The disease is highly contagious in the early stages and sexual intercourse must be avoided completely. Penicillin is curative in adequate doses but careful examination must be carried out over the following few years to ensure that the disease has been killed.

The Special Problems of Old Age

Introduction
Old age is not a sudden occurrence like puberty. It is a gradual change in the normal working of the body, a continuation of the processes that have been occurring throughout life. This change may be more rapid in some people than in others. In a healthy person, ageing seems to depend largely on genetic factors: for example, members of some families live longer than those of others.

In this section, words in italics refer to subjects that are covered by articles in the section DISEASES, SYMPTOMS AND TREATMENTS. To find these articles, turn to the index between p.54 and p.63.

The normal changes of ageing
Old age is accompanied by various changes in the body which produce slower physical reactions. There is a gradual deterioration of vision, partly due to changes in the eye lens such as *cataracts* and *long-sightedness*, and partly due to failure of the light-sensitive cells in the retina. Hearing also deteriorates, to varying degrees, due to the degeneration of the nerve cells.

Healthy senior citizens generally lead active physical lives but may find difficulty in understanding or accepting new ideas. They require almost as much food as a younger adult and need just as much sleep, although the pattern may be changed by sleeping more during the day and less at night. They usually have less stamina and find that fatigue occurs more quickly unless a regular pattern of activity is maintained.

Disease and old age
Elderly people who are healthy have good resistance to many of the common infectious illnesses, such as the common *cold* or *influenza*, because they have acquired immunity from previous infections. If, however, they do become ill it is likely to become more serious than if they were younger. It may develop into *bronchitis* or *pneumonia*, and also last longer. Immediate treatment can prevent a disease such as influenza from developing into prolonged illness.

Many physical disorders occur in old age because of the ageing of a particular organ or part of the body. An unexpected or sudden change in the physical well-being or mental alertness of an old person may be a symptom of an underlying disease. The family should not ignore this and the person should be examined by a doctor in case a treatable condition exists. Awareness and early treatment may prevent an active person from becoming incapacitated through ill-health.

The degeneration of blood vessels, due to *arteriosclerosis*, may lead to a *stroke* or a *heart attack*. In general, blood vessel diseases are made worse if the patient also has high *blood pressure* (hypertension).

Overweight people are more likely to develop *diabetes* and this may be indicated by recurrent skin and urinary infections, thirst and malaise. Hypothyroidism is another glandular disorder that may occur in old age and be associated with slow mental deterioration, physical lethargy and the danger of *hypothermia* in cold weather.

Urinary disorders are common in men because of *prostate problems* and in women because of prolapse of the womb. These may cause *incontinence* on laughing or coughing.

Arthritis is usually due to the wear and tear on joints that have been repeatedly damaged, in a minor way, throughout a hard-working life.

Two of the most common and often most difficult problems of the elderly are increasing *blindness* and *deafness*. These can be helped by the use of good lighting and adequate spectacles, and by the early use of hearing aids before deafness isolates the individual from the community.

One of the major problems of old age is loneliness. It may result from the awkwardness associated with arthritis, the shortness of breath caused by heart problems or lung disease or from the weakness following a stroke. All discourage the person from keeping active. This is particularly the case of the single person, such as a widow or widower, and leads to increasing *depression* and often to a feeling of persecution or *paranoia* that accompanies the loss of memory of the ageing mind.

Inactivity may also lead to *obesity* and frequently *constipation* from a diet consisting mainly of carbohydrates that is deficient in fresh fruit and vegetables. Constipation is commonly treated with laxatives, causing diarrhoea to alternate with periods of constipation. This, in turn, often leads to incontinence and a leakage of semi-fluid faeces which damage the skin and cause pressure sores and infection.

A cycle of mild confusion and forgetfulness, poor diet, inactivity and loneliness, constipation and diarrhoea causes a deterioration in general health. As a result, independent people can become dependent and incapable patients. This process should be prevented and the independence of the elderly maintained by intelligent help in the early stages.

Helping the confused elderly person

Confusion is one of the most characteristic problems of old age. It may result from illness, a change in surroundings, the use of new drugs for some chronic illness, or from a sudden drop in the environmental temperature. Confusion may vary from one time of the day to another. It makes the elderly argumentative, but to argue with them does not help. Talk quietly and try to change the conversation to another subject in the hope that the original one will be forgotten.

The Special Problems of Old Age

These are all problems in which early treatment is necessary to prevent further deterioration. Such treatment requires not only the co-operation of the patient but also understanding of the problems by the family and by friends. The doctor, physiotherapist or visiting nurse should be contacted to help look after the medical side of ageing but important contributions can also be made by others in terms of convenience and safety in the home. A list of useful aids and accessories is given below.

Sometimes it is necessary for the elderly to stay in hospital for a short time at the onset of a problem. This is obviously the case with a *fracture* but it may also be necessary following a *stroke* or with heart diseases in order to achieve early control of the condition. Surgery is the usual treatment for prostate problems, a prolapse, arthritis or cataracts, and may remedy the condition. Other disorders are less easily treated but may be helped by a combination of drug therapy, physiotherapy and structural alterations to the home. For example, a patient suffering from arthritis may need drugs to reduce the pain and physiotherapy to increase mobility. The nurse may use rubber mats in the bath to prevent slipping, explain how to get in and out of bed to a commode and how to use such things as wide-handled spoons and knives. A builder can be asked to level steps and put handles by the bath, by the toilet and on the staircase.

Confusion at night is more difficult to deal with as there is always the danger of falls and fractures if the confused person gets out of bed. It may help to install a baby alarm or cry-call intercom so that movements can be heard from another room. A confused person in the home puts pressure on the family and it is wise to discuss the matter with a doctor. Sometimes a short period in hospital not only helps the patient but also relieves the family of these pressures and of the associated fatigue.

Useful household aids for the elderly

A list of things which may help an old person to maintain independence and health could include some of the following suggestions.

In the bathroom: a handrail by the bath; a rail over the taps; a non-slip mat in the bath; a special seat in the bath; a handrail by the toilet; and a long-handled toothbrush.

In the bedroom: a high bed, because it is easier to get out of than a low one; a firm mattress or a board under the mattress; a commode by the bedside; a blanket support to go over the feet; and a bell by the bedside.

For clothing: self-adhesive fasteners, instead of buttons or hooks; a front-opening bra; a long-handled shoe horn; special stocking aids to help pull stockings on; slip-on shoes; non-slip soles on shoes; clip-on ties and braces.

In the kitchen: a wall can-opener; trays with non-slip surfaces and a spiked board for cutting vegetables.

For eating: unspillable cups; plate grips on the table and thickened handles on utensils (made by taping foam rubber or attaching plastic around them).

For home lighting: wall sockets placed 4ft above the floor; switches with lengthened handles; rubber balls attached to the ends of pull switches; and good reading lights.

For door handles: levers are easier to turn than knobs.

See also the section on DOMESTIC ACCIDENT PREVENTION, pp. 130-131.

Care of the elderly patient

Food. The diet should contain all the normal constituents, with adequate protein, fat and carbohydrate as well as fresh fruit and vegetables. Additional vitamins B and C, if necessary, can be given in tablet form. Sufficient fluid is essential.

Bowels. Regular bowel movements should be encouraged and only the mildest laxatives or glycerine suppositories used, and then only if necessary.

Skin care. Regular bathing or bed-bathing is important with careful drying and powdering of skin folds to prevent soreness and infection. These folds are a common site for fungal infections to occur. Hair should be brushed daily and washed once a week.

Foot care. This is very important. *Corns* and *bunions* cause pain and regular chiropody and nail clipping help to keep the older person mobile.

Teeth and gums. The mouth needs dental attention because infection and disease cause pain when eating. Some older people remove ill-fitting dentures at meal times, but this should be discouraged because it prevents normal chewing of food.

Exercise. Regular exercise helps to maintain muscle strength, joint movement and general well-being. The elderly must be encouraged to do things for themselves, to go shopping, clean the house and prepare meals.

Sleep. Drugs should be used as little as possible and only when the doctor feels they are really necessary. Drugs may cause confusion in a person who wakes during the night and may also cause sedation during the day. A warm milk drink last thing at night is an excellent sedative. Sleeping pills must never be left by the bedside.

If the person in your care is ill or bed-ridden, further valuable advice on caring for the sick at home is given in THE SICKROOM, pp. 142-143.

Care of the aged depends on maintaining their good health, giving them a real interest in life and making them feel useful to other members of the family as well as to each other.

Domestic Accident Prevention

More accidents occur in the home than anywhere else, and these are particularly likely to affect children and old people. This page lists the main danger areas and suggests how accidents may be prevented. Even when your own home is safe, remember that other houses that your children visit may not be so safe. These same safety principles also apply when you are on holiday.

Hall passage stairs
1. Well lit steps to entrances
2. No rug on a polished floor
3. Well lit stairs
4. Carpet on stairs well fixed
5. Light switches top and bottom of stairs
6. Gates at top and bottom
7. Sturdy bannister rail
8. No obstacles on the stairs

Living room
9. No trailing flex
10. Fireguard attached to wall
11. Carpets in good repair
12. No mirror over the fire

Kitchen
13. Non-slip floor
14. Cooker with firmly attached pan guards
15. Lockable cupboards for cleaning fluids
16. Cupboards out of children's reach
17. Waste disposal bin of a type that children cannot open
18. Lockable washing machine
19. CO_2 fire extinguisher

Bedroom
20. Heater that cannot burn furniture or curtains
21. Electric blanket in good order and properly earthed
22. Fire escape
23. Never smoke in bed

Nursery (child's room)
24. Cot should be high-sided and stable. No mobiles over the cot. No pillows in the cot
25. Toys should be too large for a child to put in the month
26. Safety bars on window

Bathroom
27. Handrails by bath and W.C.
28. All electric fittings should have cord switches and be placed high up, away from the bath
29. Medicine cabinet should be lockable and out of a child's reach
30. Non-slip mats on the floor and in the bath

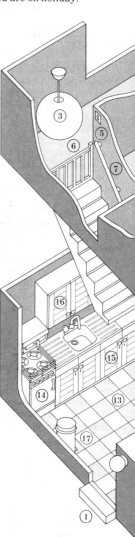

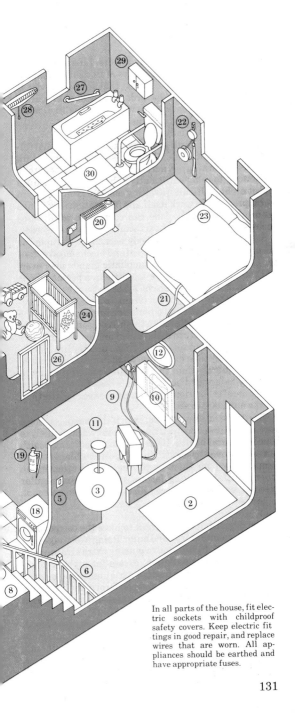

In all parts of the house, fit electric sockets with childproof safety covers. Keep electric fittings in good repair, and replace wires that are worn. All appliances should be earthed and have appropriate fuses.

131

Good Health and Body Maintenance

Good health depends on many factors. Lifestyle, eating habits, the use of drugs and ways of relaxation may all affect general health. In the text that follows, advice is offered about common hazards to health that can be avoided and suggests ways in which the health of mind and body can best be maintained.

The causes of ill health

People who work hard and competitively for personal fulfilment or financial gain lead stressful lives. In certain cases their working day may be so full of tension that they are unable to relax sufficiently at home in the evenings and at night. Difficult travelling conditions on the way to work, pressure in work itself and frustration if work has been unsatisfactorily done can contribute to illnesses such as a stomach ulcer, heart attack or nervous disorder.

Stress is harmful to the body because it disrupts the normal patterns of physiological and biochemical activity. Certain endocrine and lymphatic glands may overwork and others may work too little in a person who is under stress. The digestive system, particularly the stomach, reacts poorly to variations in metabolic requirements and the heart and circulation are damaged by the excessive demands placed on them. A person living under stress is more likely to make use of artificial stimulants and sedatives than someone living a quieter life. Such a person is likely to be more interested in meals that can be prepared quickly than in foods that constitute a more correctly balanced diet. Someone whose lifestyle allows little time of relaxation is also likely to have too little time to take adequate exercise.

Clarifying one's priorities, even if this means taking a less aggressive or competitive stance at work, is likely to benefit general health. If the job is too important, health can be improved by identifying the potential dangers and compensating for them by paying special attention to other health-improving factors such as taking regular exercise, eating a balanced diet, and avoiding alcohol, tobacco and other drugs.

Diet

For good health it is important to have the correct body weight for your age, sex and build. Being overweight is a proven hazard. In addition to putting extra strain on the joints, heart and circulation, excess fat probably indicates that too much rich food (which is high in cholesterol) is being eaten. A high level of cholesterol in the blood may cause deterioration of the arteries and so increase the risk of thrombosis.

A healthy diet must contain a variety of types of food. Carbohydrates, proteins, fats, vitamins and minerals are required in varying proportions. Vitamins and minerals are essential but are only required in minute quantities. Fats give the most energy but they may also cause ill health through blood vessel disease. Proteins are necessary for growth and the basic protein elements (amino acids) may be obtained from many foods including cereals, vegetables and nuts. A varied diet ensures that all the necessary amino acids are present. Carbohydrates occur in various forms and are the basis of most people's diet. They are primarily a source of energy but some types of carbohydrate also form the roughage (fibre bulk) that is required if the bowel muscles are to function properly.

Eating a balanced diet is essential to any programme for maintaining good health. Most people eat too much and many eat the wrong things. It is probable that if the diet is restricted to those foods that are best suited to the body's requirements, the desire to overeat disappears. Sugar (a carbohydrate) and animal fats should be avoided as much as possible. Unsweetened fruit juices, water and bulky fibre foods are generally beneficial. Starch (also a carbohydrate), which is the chief constituent of potatoes and bread, is a necessary part of any diet and a moderate intake of starchy carbohydrate will not lead to obesity. Many of the nutritional components of potatoes and other vegetables are found in their skins. The whole grain of wheat that is used in wholemeal bread is more nutritious than the refined flour used to make white bread and this should be remembered if bread and potatoes make up a large part of the diet.

The small quantities of essential vitamins and minerals that the body requires are provided by most diets that contain a variety of foods such as vegetables, milk, eggs, fruit and meat. If vegetables are boiled some vitamins are destroyed by heat, or lost because they are water-soluble. In affluent countries many foods contain additional vitamins and for this reason ill health due to vitamin deficiency is rare. A deficiency of iron does sometimes occur in women because of heavy menstruation. If this occurs, listlessness and other symptoms of iron-deficiency anaemia may appear. It has been suggested that large quantities of some vitamins, particularly vitamin C, may help to prevent, and may speed recovery from, illness but at present scientific opinion is divided on this question.

The types of dietary fats that are potentially harmful include the saturated fats and cholesterol. The term saturated refers to the chemical structure of the fat molecules. The degrees of saturation are relative. Most animal fats are saturated and typically appear solid when cold. Unsaturated fats are obtained primarily from plants and fish and are usually liquid. Cholesterol is produced by the human body and is necessary for the formation of new tissues but an excess of cholesterol in the blood leads to it being deposited in the walls of arteries and damaging these vessels.

Good Health and Body Maintenance

Obesity is a serious hazard to health. In an older person it can be as dangerous as regular smoking. The appearance of loose fatty flesh around the face, upper arms, chest, waist or thighs is the most obvious indication of obesity. A table of ideal weights may also prove useful provided that natural variations such as sex, build and age are taken into account. The table below estimates the ideal naked weight of a 30-year-old person of average build. A person of heavy or light build should add or subtract seven pounds from the weight given and anyone between the ages of 20 and 45 should add or subtract a pound for each year that they are older or younger than 30. The table covers a middle range of heights and anyone not covered by this range should add or subtract four pounds for each inch of difference.

Height	feet	5'3"	5'4"	5'5"	5'6"	5'7"	5'8"	5'9"	5'10"	5'11"	6'0"
	cm	160	163	165	168	170	173	175	178	180	183
Male	lb	135	139	143	147	151	155	159	163	167	171
Weight	kg	61.2	63.0	64.9	66.7	68.5	70.3	72.1	73.9	75.7	77.6
Female	lb	126	130	134	138	142	146	150	154	158	162
Weight	kg	57.1	59.0	60.9	62.6	64.4	66.2	68.0	69.8	71.7	73.5

No table of this kind can do more than offer a rough guide to the correct weight of a person who has a particular height and build but in general it may be assumed that anyone who differs from the weight calculated from this table by more than seven pounds is probably over- or underweight. Such a person should consult a doctor for further advice.

If you need to lose weight, ask your doctor for advice about a suitable diet that takes into account any medical problems you may have and that supplements any nutrients that may be lacking.

In nearly all cases the body puts on fat because the amount of food eaten is greater than the amount of energy being used up. The basis of any successful slimming programme is the correct balance between the intake and the output of energy. The easiest way an overweight person can improve this balance is to eat less and to take more exercise. It is also important to be selective in the choice of food because the energy obtained from some foods (such as fats) is so much greater than from others (such as proteins) that fewer of the high-energy foods are required.

Exercise

Regular exercise is essential for good health and is particularly important for preventing heart and lung disorders. It increases physical strength, suppleness and stamina, and often encourages mental alertness as well as physical agility. Exercise also improves the complexion and gives confidence in posture and movement.

A systematic programme of physical exercise should not be too ambitious initially. A ten-minute jog each day, just fast enough to produce breathlessnes and to increase the pulse rate without strain, brings about a dramatic improvement in the health of most people, especially those who have sedentary jobs. Jogging can easily be combined with other daily obligations such as walking the dog or returning home after taking the children to nursery school. As an alternative to jogging, a game such as tennis or badminton, or swimming at least twice a week, also helps to maintain physical fitness in ways that are pleasant and do not require a large amount of self-discipline. Specific exercises are particularly valuable for improving the strength and shape of specific parts of the body. Exercising the abdominal muscles helps to reduce stomach fat. Running or step-up exercises strengthen the legs. Exercising the muscles of the waist gives the waist a better shape. These exercises can be developed from the range of warm-up exercises that are used by athletes to prepare their muscles for strenuous activity.

People who take little exercise may find that their muscles and joints lose suppleness and strength. For such people exercising neck, shoulder, arm, chest, back, waist, hip, leg and ankle muscles for a few minutes each day will greatly improve the feeling of general physical health.

Relaxation

In addition to taking regular exercise many people also need to learn how to relax. One of the best ways of relaxing is to develop an interest or hobby outside the contexts of work and family. Such interests are relaxing because they distract from the pressures of life without necessarily creating stressful demands themselves.

There is more to relaxing than simply getting enough sleep and physical rest and in general it is probably true to say that the mental aspects of relaxation are even more important than the physical. Hobbies and holidays alone are not enough to solve the problem for many people, especially if there are persistent causes of anxiety. For this and other reasons the use of mental or spiritual exercises such as meditation to aid relaxation is becoming increasingly common. There are many schools of meditation and these advocate different techniques in order to achieve the desired states of relaxation or spiritual peace. Another Eastern discipline that is popular in the West is yoga, which is often found to be particularly valuable because of the ways in which it combines exercises to relieve physical tension with techniques that help to relieve mental stress.

This section has suggested how good health can be encouraged and maintained. More detailed advice on these topics can be obtained from a doctor and specialists in the appropriate field can also be consulted.

The Sickroom

Caring for someone recovering from an illness, an old person or a member of the family who may be ill for some time can be made more pleasant for the sick (as well as for the healthy) if the patient can be cared for at home. The sickroom may be the patient's own bedroom or another more convenient room in the house. Whichever room is chosen, there are certain basic requirements and many helpful techniques that can contribute to the comfort of the patient, to the convenience of the nurse and to the general well-being of the whole household.

Basic requirements

The basic requirements of a sickroom are a comfortable bed with a firm mattress; additional pillows; and a well-ventilated room at a comfortable temperature. A non-slip floor will also help. Remove any rugs from beside the bed. Put a chair near the bed, as an aid to getting out of bed and for the patient to sit on if necessary.

The bedside table should have a jug of water and a glass, a hand-bell or electric bell for the patient to call for help if necessary, and a reading light that can be dimmed at night. There should be a toilet near by and there should also be a vomit bowl if necessary.

Taking a temperature: mouth

Shake the thermometer so that the reading is below minimum on the scale and place the thermometer under the patient's tongue. Ask the patient to close the lips around the thermometer and leave it there for at least two minutes. Remove the thermometer, read the mercury level and write down the reading. Shake the thermometer so that the mercury level falls below minimum again. Clean the bulb with antiseptic before putting it away in its case.

Taking a temperature: rectum

This method is generally used for babies. Grease the end of the thermometer with petroleum jelly. Lay the baby on its back, hold its feet in the air, and insert the bulb of the thermometer just inside the rectum. Leave it in place for at least two minutes. Remove the thermometer, read the temperature and write down the reading. The rectal temperature is usually about 1° higher than the temperature taken in the mouth.

Diet and fluids

A feverish patient requires more fluid than usual and must be encouraged to drink at least four pints of liquid a day. Solid food can be a problem because most bed-ridden patients have a poor appetite. Food should be appetizing and nutritious and small portions should be given.

Vomiting

To help someone who is vomiting, support the forehead with one hand and hold a bowl in the other. When vomiting has ceased, sponge the patient's face and forehead with cool water and rinse the patient's mouth.

Drugs

Drugs must be kept away from the patient's reach to prevent accidental overdosage. They must only be given as directed by the doctor.

Giving a bed bath

The key principle is to wash one part of the patient at a time and keep the rest of the body covered with a thick towel or a blanket to prevent the patient getting cold. The sequence should be:
1. Put a large towel under the patient, then cover the patient and wash and dry the face and neck. 2. Wash and dry each arm and the adjacent side of the chest, completing one side before starting the other. 3. Cover the chest and arms before washing and drying the abdomen and groin. 4. Wash each leg, keeping the rest of the body covered. 5. Roll the patient onto the side and wash the back. Throughout washing it is important to dry the skin thoroughly and to powder creases, particularly under the breasts, in the groin and between the buttocks.

Care of the mouth

The patient should rinse the mouth with a mouth wash after meals and brush the teeth at least twice a day. False teeth must be cleaned regularly. Dry lips should be moistened with a lip salve.

Care of hair and nails

Hair should be brushed and combed at least twice a day. Nails must be kept clean and cut regularly.

Humidity

The sickroom should not be too dry, because dry air may aggravate coughing or cause discomfort to breathing. Humidity may be increased by leaving large bowls of water in the room, or by boiling a kettle in the room (away from the bed).

Blanket supports

Blanket supports are used to take the weight of the bedclothes off the patient's legs. A temporary support can be made by using a stool on its side and inserting its lower legs under the mattress.

Nose drops

Make sure the patient is sitting or lying comfortably with the head tilted back. Draw up liquid in a dropper and insert the dropper into a nostril. Release the number of drops prescribed and repeat in the other nostril. Ask the patient to sniff to inhale the drops.

Eye drops

Make sure the patient is sitting or lying comfortably with the head tilted back. Stand behind and with one hand pull the lower eyelid gently downwards. Rest the other hand, holding the dropper, on the patient's forehead. Insert the drops exactly as prescribed between the eye and the lowered lid. Repeat into the other eye. Ask the patient to blink several times.

Keeping Healthy on Holiday

When going on holiday, and particularly when travelling abroad, certain precautions help to ensure that problems of ill health do not arise or that, if they do, they are prevented from becoming serious.

General advice

Health insurance should be adequate to cover the possibility of hospitalization. If you suffer from any recurrent or permanent medical problem, or if you are taking a young child abroad, discuss specific precautions with your doctor before you depart. The advice of an experienced authority should also be sought if you intend to visit the tropics. A phrase book that gives the foreign names of illnesses and symptoms may also prove useful.

Take great care when sunbathing until you are fully acclimatized. At first, lie in the sun for only 10 minutes in the morning and 10 in the late afternoon. Increase this by 10 minutes a day until you are tanned but not burned. Do not lie in the sun during the hottest part of the day.

Avoid unwashed fruit, cooked foods that have been allowed to cool, and unsterilized water, because any of these may carry infectious organisms that can cause food poisoning. Do not swim within two hours of eating a meal because the exercise and the temperature of the water may lead to cramps if the stomach is still in the process of digesting food.

Animals

When away from home and particularly when travelling abroad, avoid contact with all animals and never allow children to touch or fondle them. Several dangerous diseases, including rabies, may be carried in the saliva, in the faeces or on the skin of domestic animals.

Medicaments

A list of basic preparations to take on holiday should include sunburn lotion, insect-repellent cream, salt tablets, body powder and aspirin. Anti-diarrhoeal drugs such as Lomotil and kaolin mixture may also be useful. A pair of scissors, a roll of sticking plaster and some antiseptic cream or antibiotic powder should be included.

Immunization

If you are travelling in a region where malaria is endemic, you should take antimalarial drugs such as chloroquine, Daraprim or Paludrine for a week before and for a month after, as well as during, your visit. International certificates of vaccination against smallpox, cholera, yellow fever, and sometimes typhus and plague are required by many countries. Check also that existing certificates are not out of date. Travellers outside Western Europe and North America should also be immunized against poliomyelitis, typhoid (TAB), tetanus and infectious hepatitis.

Any illness that develops shortly after your return from abroad should be reported to a doctor.

Medicines to Keep in the Home

Keep a stock of medicines and basic accessories in a safe place, ideally in a separate cupboard, that is well out of the reach of children. Fit the cupboard with a childproof lock and do not use it to store anything except things for medical use.

The cupboard should contain all medicines prescribed by a doctor. Pills should never be left by the bedside where children may help themselves. Throw away all medicines that are no longer being used.

The medicine cupboard should contain:

Emergency information, including the telephone
    numbers of your local doctor, hospital and chemist;
large, blunt-ended scissors;
square-ended tweezers for removing splinters;
clinical thermometer in its case;
packet of safety pins;
packet of cotton wool;
two 2 in (5 cm) elastic (crepe) bandages;
two 3 in (7.5 cm) elastic (crepe) bandages;
five sterile gauze dressings in individual packets;
two non-adherent sterile dressings with perforated
    plastic film to be used on burns and grazes;
elastic adhesive bandage 4 in (10 cm) wide;
adhesive dressing strip with central medicated gauze;
packet or box of individual adhesive plasters;
sterile eye pad;
two rolls of non-allergic surgical tape, 1 in (2.5 cm) wide.

The following drugs may also be useful for:

colds:	chlorpheniramine tablets (Piriton); ephedrine nose drops (10 ml bottle);
constipation:	bisacodyl tablets (Dulcolax; glycerine suppositories (pack of 10);
coughs:	proprietary cough mixture;
fever:	soluble aspirin tablets (300 mg);
diarrhoea:	kaolin mixture (200 ml);
grazes:	cetrimide cream (Savlon);
headaches and pain	codeine and paracetamol tablets (bottle of 25);
indigestion:	magnesium trisilicate mixture (200 ml bottle);
rash and sunburn:	calamine lotion (200 ml bottle);
sore throat:	benzalkonium lozenges (pack of 25); glycerine and thymol mouth wash (200 ml bottle);
wound cleaning:	hexachlorophane solution (200 ml bottle).

In addition to these, some medicines are available in special preparations for children.

Introduction to Medicinal Drugs

Treatment with drugs is one of the most important aspects of modern medicine but it is also one of the areas of medicine about which the lay person knows least. Progress in the science of drug therapy has led to the development of thousands of different drugs, many of which are used specifically to combat particular illnesses or specific disease-causing organisms. For practical purposes these different drugs are classified into types, according to their functions or general characteristics and some of the important features of these types are described in the following pages.

Anaesthetics
General anaesthetics are given before major surgery is carried out. A premedication injection is usually given before a general anaesthetic. It acts as a relaxant with a mild sedative effect; it also dries the mouth. Local anaesthetics may be injected, to numb a nerve or an area of skin, or sprayed or applied locally to the area to be anaesthetized. Occasionally an allergic reaction may occur.

Antacids
Antacids may be alkalis used to neutralize stomach acids or drugs that reduce stomach acid secretion. Some preparations combine both sorts. Overdosage may cause a dry mouth and drowsiness.

Anti-allergic drugs
These are the antihistamines, corticosteroid drugs and sodium cromoglycate (Intal). These can be used in eye drops, in nasal and bronchial sprays, or as powders that are inhaled.

Antibiotics
Antibiotics comprise several groups of drugs that can kill bacteria. The use of antibiotics, however, may be hazardous. Excessive use of antibiotics encourages the development of resistant strains of bacteria and may also lead to an increased likelihood of allergic reactions. Particular infections often require specific antibiotics. Some of the more toxic antibiotics are safe to use on the skin but should not be taken internally.

Anticoagulants
Anticoagulants are drugs that interfere with the normal clotting of the blood and reduce the chances of thrombosis. They are used after deep vein and coronary thrombosis and in some forms of heart and gynaecological surgery in which the hazards of venous and arterial thrombosis are increased.

Anticonvulsant drugs
Anticonvulsants control epilepsy, and treatment with them usually continues for many years. Occasionally allergic reactions occur but, on the whole, these drugs are considered safe.

Antidepressants

Antidepressants work within the brain to alter the patient's mood. They may take two to three weeks to produce an effect, and the course of treatment should continue for several weeks after this. Apart from stimulant drugs (see *Stimulants*, below), such as amphetamine, there are two main groups of antidepressants. One group, the tricyclic antidepressants, benefits those who wake too early and suffer depression and anxiety at the beginning of the day. These may also cause dryness in the mouth, constipation and slight drowsiness. The other group, the mono-amine oxidase inhibitors (MAOI), may help those who sleep normally but suffer depression all day. This group of drugs may cause adverse reactions to certain foods such as cheese, yeast or meat extracts, broad beans, yogurt, alcohol and sometimes to other drugs, particularly pain-killers. Tranquillizers are often used in combination with antidepressants because anxiety is frequently associated with depression.

Anti-diabetic drugs

Anti-diabetic drugs are taken to replace or to stimulate the production of insulin. Excessive amounts may cause faintness, dizziness and sometimes coma due to hypoglycaemia. Insulin is the most common drug used in the treatment of severe diabetes but can be given only by injection. It is prepared from the pancreas of pigs or cattle and in rare cases this may cause an allergic reaction. Simple preparations or slow release preparations act for varying lengths of time. The dose has to be carefully calculated, according to the patient's requirements.

Anti-diarrhoeal drugs

The most common preparation used to treat diarrhoea is kaolin which is sometimes combined with a small amount of morphine. The morphine group, including codeine, has a direct constipating effect on the bowel. Some types of antispasmodic drug (see *Antispasmodic drugs*, below) may be obtained on prescription and these are frequently used by holidaymakers to control traveller's diarrhoea. Antibiotics may be used in some severe infections.

Antifungal drugs

Antifungal drugs are used in the treatment of moniliasis and tinea infections such as thrush and athlete's foot. Antifungals are usually applied directly to the affected area or membranes as creams, ointments or pessaries.

Antihistamines

This group of drugs is used in the treatment of allergies, asthma, insect bites and urticaria. They also act to prevent motion sickness and may be used as sedatives for children. They occasionally cause unexpected stimulation or over-sedation and can be dangerous if taken before driving or using machinery. They can cause serious drowsiness if taken at the same time as alcohol.

Introduction to Medicinal Drugs

Antimalarial drugs

Antimalarial drugs must be taken regularly when entering a malarious region and their use must be continued for at least a month after leaving the area. Different types of antimalarial are designed to be taken either daily or weekly, depending on the kind of drug. If the disease is caught, specific drugs such as quinine or chloroquine may be required.

Anti-nausea and anti-emetic drugs

Antihistamines and many of the major tranquillizer drugs have anti-nausea effects. Their use is not to be recommended during pregnancy because they may cause fetal damage. Particular care should be used if they are taken when driving. Alcohol should not be consumed when taking these drugs.

Anti-Parkinsonian drugs

These include levodopa and related drugs that have been of major benefit in treating Parkinson's disease, but if given in large doses they may cause nausea, faintness and weakness as additional side-effects.

Anti-rheumatic drugs

Mild anti-rheumatics include aspirin and similar preparations. Strong anti-rheumatic drugs include those based on phenylbutazone and indomethacin which are effective but often cause peptic ulcers and blood disorders. Occasionally injections of gold salts and other drugs are used. Pain-killing drugs are often used in combination with anti-rheumatic drugs in the treatment of arthritic disorders. In certain cases cortisone and other steroids may be required.

Antispasmodic drugs

These drugs relax smooth muscle in the intestine and the lungs. Intestinal antispasmodics can be given in the form of tablets or injections to relieve diarrhoea or colic. Antispasmodics for the lungs are often called bronchodilators and can be given as tablets or they can be inhaled. They are used particularly in the treatment of types of asthma.

Anti-viral drugs

There are relatively few anti-viral drugs. Some are used in the treatment of shingles, cold sores and virus infections of the eye. Others are used in treating smallpox. Research is currently in progress to develop anti-viral drugs that may help to combat influenza.

Corticosteroid drugs

Corticosteroids are synthesized as cortisol or as chemical modifications of it to increase its effective strength. They prevent the body reacting to internal or external irritants and diseases by interfering with the body's normal reactions to infection and by reducing inflammation. The drugs can be used in the form of eye and ear preparations; in nose drops and sprays, in the treatment of asthma; and in other different forms such as creams, to treat such skin conditions as eczema and psoriasis. Injections of corticosteroids are sometimes given directly into joints in certain forms of arthritis. Corticosteroid drugs taken by mouth will prevent the adrenal gland reacting to the stress of accidents, illnesses or surgery and this effect will persist for some months after the dosage of the drug has been stopped. Large amounts, taken over a long time, may cause a loss of calcium from the bones, an increase in weight, abnormal skin markings and a roundness in the shape of the face.

Cytotoxic drugs

These drugs destroy cell tissue and are used in the chemical treatment (chemotherapy) of cancer.

Diuretics

Diuretics increase the loss of water and salts through the kidneys. They are often used to treat heart diseases and some forms of kidney disease. Additional potassium salts should be given with some preparations, if they are used for any length of time, to prevent muscle weakness.

Heart and blood pressure drugs

Digoxin is used in heart failure and in cases of tachycardia (rapid heart beat) to increase the strength of the heart muscle and to reduce the pulse rate. Blood pressure can be reduced by a variety of drugs, including diuretics and the beta-adrenergic blocking agents that work by preventing the action of adrenalin.

Hormones

Adrenalin is used to treat severe allergic reactions (anaphylaxis) and severe asthma. It causes palpitations, sweating and a sense of anxiety. It may also be used as a heart stimulant. Thyroid hormone (thyroxine) is used in the treatment of hypothyroidism (myxoedema). Preparations from the pituitary gland, for example vasopressin, the antidiuretic hormone, are used to stimulate the contraction of blood vessels. Female sex hormones, such as oestrogen, are used in the treatment of menstrual disorders, in the contraceptive pill and in treating cancer of the prostate gland in men. Male hormones, known as androgens, and synthetic preparations are used to increase body strength after a debilitating illness.

Hypnotic and sedative drugs

These are used to treat insomnia. The barbiturate group are potentially addictive and may be fatal in overdosage. All these drugs tend to reduce dreaming and when they are stopped a period of 1 to 2 weeks of lighter sleep and of increased dreaming commonly occurs.

Laxatives

Laxatives stimulate bowel function. There are three main groups. Some act by increasing the bulk of the faeces, either by adding insoluble salts or non-digestible vegetable fibre. Others soften and lubricate faeces. The third group stimulates bowel wall contractions.

143

Introduction to Medicinal Drugs

Pain-killing drugs

Mild pain-killers are based on aspirin and similar drugs. Occasionally they may cause skin rashes or intestinal bleeding, particularly if used to excess. Moderate pain-killers are based on codeine and similar chemicals. Their most common side-effect is constipation. Strong pain-killers such as morphine are derived from the opiate group. These drugs are sedative and addictive but are useful after operations and accidents or in the treatment of advanced cancer, when the relief of pain is more important than avoiding possible side-effects.

Tranquillizers

Minor hypnotics and sedatives used in small amounts act as tranquillizers. The benzodiazepines (Valium, Librium, etc) are frequently used in the treatment of anxiety. They are also used with antidepressant drugs. They seldom cause adverse reactions apart from giving an artificial sense of elation and sometimes drowsiness. It is dangerous to drink alcohol when taking these drugs. Their most harmful side-effect is the sense of psychological dependence they may encourage. Major tranquillizers often have an anti-nausea and sedative effect. They are used in mental illnesses such as schizophrenia and alcoholism. Occasionally they cause liver damage.

Vaccines

Vaccines are used to create immunity and so are used to protect the body against infections. They are commonly made from a killed or weakened variety of the organism which causes the disease. Babies and children should be protected by vaccination against diphtheria, whooping cough, tetanus, poliomyelitis, measles, German measles (rubella) and tuberculosis. Vaccination against smallpox and injections to protect against cholera and yellow fever have to be given to travellers before they visit certain areas of the world where these diseases exist. Typhoid, typhus and plague vaccines are also available and may also be required by immigration authorities in some countries. Travellers should be vaccinated before they leave their home country.

Vaso-constrictive drugs

These are used to cause blood vessels to contract. Adrenalin is sometimes used in cases of severe shock to raise the patient's blood pressure. Ergotamine is used in some anti-migraine preparations but it should only be taken at the onset of symptoms. Excessive use of ergotamine may cause vomiting.

Vaso-dilator drugs

Vaso-dilators are used to expand blood vessels. They are used in angina pectoris to relieve or prevent heart pain and are usually prepared in a form that can be inhaled, chewed or swallowed. On exercise they may cause palpitations and flushing.

Family medical history

Name				
Date of birth				
National insurance no.				
Blood group				
Allergies				
Regular medication				
Serious past illnesses				
Next medical check-up				
Most recent X-ray				